Electro

Handbook of
Electrogastrography

KENNETH L. KOCH
ROBERT M. STERN

OXFORD
UNIVERSITY PRESS
2004

OXFORD
UNIVERSITY PRESS

Oxford New York
Auckland   Bangkok   Buenos Aires   Cape Town   Chennai
Dar es Salaam   Delhi   Hong Kong   Istanbul   Karachi   Kolkata
Kuala Lumpur   Madrid   Melbourne   Mexico City   Mumbai
Nairobi   São Paulo   Shanghai   Taipei   Tokyo   Toronto

Published by Oxford University Press, Inc.
198 Madison Avenue, New York, New York 10016
www.oup.com

Library of Congress Cataloging-in-Publication Data
Handbook of electrogastrography /
by Kenneth L. Koch and Robert M. Stern.
p. cm.   Includes bibliographical references and index.
ISBN 0-19-514788-X
1. Electrogastrography.
I. Koch, Kenneth L. II. Stern, Robert Morris, 1937–
RC804.E4 H36 2003   616.3'307547—dc21   2003002110

1 2 3 4 5 6 7 8 9

Printed in the United States of America
on acid-free paper

Preface

....

Electrogastrography refers to the methods of recording electrogastrograms (EGGs). EGG rhythms reflect the gastric pacesetter potentials or slow waves of the stomach. Pacesetter potentials are crucial electrical depolarization and repolarization waves because they control the timing and propagation velocity of gastric peristaltic contractions. Gastric peristaltic contractions are responsible for mixing and emptying the foodstuffs that are ingested throughout the day. In humans, the gastric pacesetter potential is approximately 3 cycles per minute (cpm). Thus, the 3-cpm EGG signals are noninvasive recordings of the electrical activity of the stomach in health.

During the past 20 years, there have been important advances in the understanding of stomach electrical and contractile activity. It has also become clear that the normal electrical rhythm of the stomach may become very disordered. *Gastric dysrhythmias* are abnormalities of gastric myoelectrical activity. These disturbed electrical rhythms are recorded in the EGG signal. Abnormally fast electrical rhythm are termed *tachygastrias*, and abnormally slow rhythms are described as *bradygastrias*. Gastric dysrhythmias are common in the clinical settings of nausea that occur during motion sickness, chemotherapy, and the nausea of pregnancy. Gastric dysrhythmias are frequently present in patients with functional dyspepsia, unexplained nausea, and diabetic, idiopathic, and postsurgical gastroparesis. Furthermore, correction of gastric dysrhythmias with drug therapies or electrical stimulation is associated with improvement in nausea and vomiting. In many respects, the recording of the EGG is analogous to the recording of electrocardiogram. Thus, there has been increasing interest in electrogastrography and in the diagnostic value of EGG patterns.

The purpose of this handbook is to present the physiological basis for electrogastrography with a series of diagrams, illustrations, and examples of actual EGGs and analyses. The authors have more than 60 years of combined experiences in evaluating patients with a wide variety of nausea and vomiting syndromes and in studying healthy subjects in a variety of psychophysiological experiments. Thousands of EGG recordings have been recorded and studied by the authors. The EGGs were recorded from diverse patients ranging from diabetic patients with gastroparesis to patients with dysmotility-like dyspepsia symptoms and unexplained nausea. EGGs from healthy subjects who became nauseous in various controlled studies are also described. The handbook is not meant to be an exhaustive treatise on electrogastrography. Rather than reviewing the contributions of many investigators, the handbook describes the practical aspects of how to record excellent EGGs and the methods available for analyzing, quantifying, and interpreting the EGG recordings. The authors also acknowledge the work of Kent Sanders and colleagues who contributed chapter 2 on the basic electrical properties of the stomach.

With increasing interest in the EGG from researchers and clinicians, this book should become a helpful reference for the interpretation of normal and abnormal EGG recordings. An EGG recording device and software analysis system have been cleared by the Food and Drug Administration and are available commercially. One of the authors (K. L. Koch) has a financial interest in the company that manufactures this medical equipment. The EGG is a unique and noninvasive diagnostic test for gastroenterologists in multidisciplinary group practices, in clinical gastrointestinal motility centers, and in research laboratories. EGG recordings will be of interest to internists and family medicine physicians who treat patients with dyspepsia or gastric dysfunction. Diabetologists may have a particular interest in EGG patterns in patients with dyspepsia symptoms and type 1 or 2 diabetes. Relationships among gastric neuromuscular function, plasma glucose levels, and insulin therapy are becoming more appreciated and integrated into diabetes care. The handbook will also be a reference source for fellows in gastroenterology and researchers with an interest in gastric myoelectrical activity. In addition, we hope the handbook will serve as a primer for researchers in fields such as psychosomatic medicine and psychophysiology who are in need of a noninvasive method for quantifying gastric myoelectrical activity.

Winston-Salem, North Carolina   K. L. K.
University Park, Pennsylvania   R. M. S.

Acknowledgments

....

The authors gratefully acknowledge the excellent secretarial assistance of Mrs. Pamela Bohn and the expert medical illustration efforts of Ms. Marty Hansell.

Contents

Contributors

....

Kenneth L. Koch, M.D.
Section of Gastroenterology and Hepatology
Wake Forest University Baptist Medical Center
Wake Forest University
Winston-Salem, North Carolina

Robert M. Stern, Ph.D.
Psychology Department
The Pennsylvania State University
University Park, Pennsylvania

**Kenton M. Sanders, Ph.D., Tamas Ördög, Ph.D.,
Sang Don Koh, Ph.D., Sean M. Ward, Ph.D.**
Department of Physiology and Cell Biology
University of Nevada School of Medicine
Reno, Nevada

Handbook of
Electrogastrography

1

Brief History of Electrogastrography

During the first half of the twentieth century, before the availability of computerized literature searches, scientists who were working independently often discovered similar measures, phenomena, or relationships. The electrogastrogram (EGG) was discovered independently by at least three investigators: Walter Alvarez, a gastroenterologist; I. Harrison Tumpeer, a pediatrician; and R. C. Davis, a psychophysiologist.

On October 14, 1921, after considerable experimentation with rabbits at the University of California in San Francisco, Walter Alvarez[1] recorded the first human EGG. Figure 1.1 shows this EGG, which was recorded from an elderly woman with an abdominal wall hernia. The woman was so thin that Alvarez could observe gastric contractions of 3 min in the upper abdomen that corresponded to the 3 cycles/min (cpm) electrical waves that are clearly seen in the EGG recording. Alvarez did not publish additional studies with the EGG during his long and productive career, probably because of the technical difficulties inherent in recording such a weak signal before the development of good vacuum tube amplifiers.

1

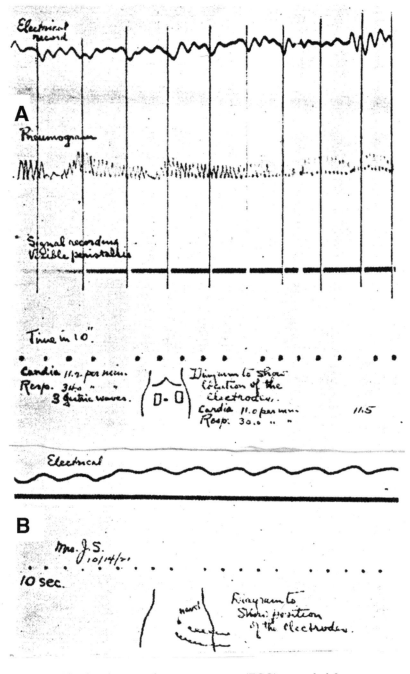

Figure 1.1. The first human electrogastrogram (EGG) recorded from a woman whose abdominal wall was so thin that her gastric peristalsis was easily visible. (*A*) EGG (top tracing), respiration, and markers indicating when visible peristalsis was observed. Note the temporal correspondence between the EGG signal and these markers. (*B*) EGG (the tracing just above the horizontal line) from a different electrode placement that is shown in the figure. (Reprinted with permission from Alvarez, 1922.)

I. Harrison Tumpeer, a pediatrician working at Michael Reese Hospital in Chicago, reported in 1926[2] that while he was attempting to record the EGG, "Alvarez of California published his results." In a subsequent publication,[3] Tumpeer successfully recorded the EGG from a 5-week-old child who had pyloric stenosis. Tumpeer and his coworkers selected this particular subject because they could observe gastric contractions by simply watching the surface of the skin over the abdomen. Figure 1.2 shows a portion of this EGG. Tumpeer described the EGG as looking like an electrocardiogram (ECG) with a slowly changing baseline. Tumpeer mentioned that cardiologists in 1926 often noted a changing baseline in ECG recordings that they could not explain. Thus, the EGG had been recorded, but perhaps not recognized as such, since the time of the first ECG at the turn of the twentieth century. Tumpeer used limb leads to record his EGG (not abdominal leads) because of his concern that each gastric contraction caused physical displacement of the skin over the child's abdomen. Subsequent studies[4] showed that simultaneous recordings from limbs and abdomen are similar except that the amplitude of the EGG is greatly reduced from recordings from the limb leads.

R. C. Davis, a psychophysiologist, began a series of exploratory studies with the EGG in the mid-1950s. Because he was not aware of the earlier EGG work of Alvarez or Tumpeer, he was the third person to independently discover the EGG. Davis was primarily interested in the interactive effects of psychological and physiological factors on gastric functioning. Davis and colleagues published two papers on the EGG before his untimely death in 1961, papers that stimulated several other investigators to begin conducting EGG research.

In 1957, Davis and coworkers[5] described their attempt to validate the EGG using simultaneous recordings from needle electrodes, a mine detector that picked up the movements of a steel ball in the subject's gastrointestinal tract, and the EGG. They used needle electrodes that were insulated except at the tip so that they could rule out cutaneous tissue as the source of the EGG signal. Figure 1.3 shows a portion of one such simultaneous recording from Davis' laboratory.

In 1959, Davis and his coworkers[6] described validation studies of the EGG using swallowed balloons; Figure 1.4 shows simultaneous records obtained from EGG surface electrodes and an intragastric balloon, showing correspondence between the EGG recording from the upper left quadrant of the abdomen (top tracing) and the recording from the balloon (bottom tracing). In this same study,

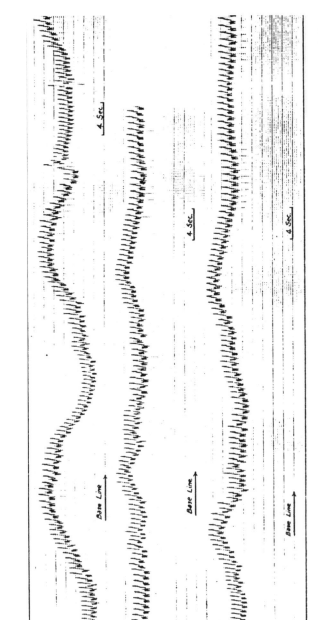

Figure 1.2. Electrocardiogram recorded with limb lead III from an infant with pyloric stenosis. The authors reported that the 20-second wavelike shifts in the tracings corresponded to visible gastric peristaltic waves. Subsequent radiological examination of the child revealed obstruction caused by a pyloric tumor. (Reprinted with permission from Tumpeer and Phillips, 1932.)

Needle   (a)

EGG   (b)

Mine
Detector   (c)

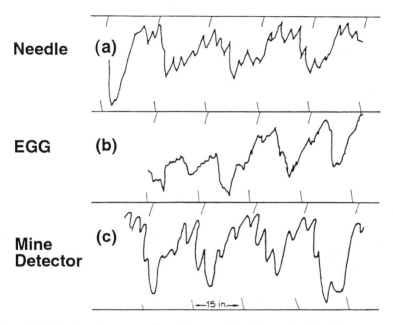

|←—15 in.—→|

Figure 1.3. Simultaneous recordings from needle electrodes (*a*), electrogastro-gram (EGG) (*b*), and mine detector (*c*). The needle electrodes were insulated except at the tip to prevent the recording of galvanic skin responses; one was in-serted in the skin of the abdomen and the other in the subject's arm. The EGG electrodes were both placed on the surface of the abdomen. The mine detector tracing was made by having the subject swallow a metal ball and then tracking its movement with a mine detector. Note the similarity in 3-cpm waves in the three records and the baseline shift in the EGG recording. "15 in" indicates 15 sec-onds. See text for details. (Reprinted with permission from Davis, Garafolo, and Gault, 1957.)

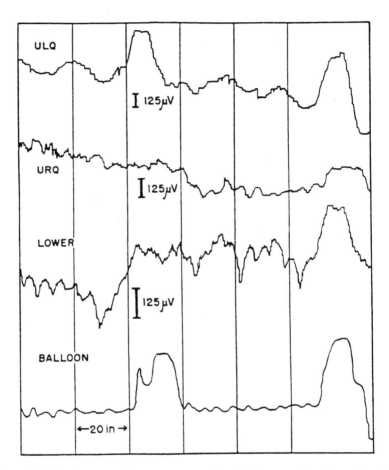

Figure 1.4. Simultaneous electrogastrographic (EGG) recordings from three locations and from an intragastric balloon. The top three tracings are EGGs from the upper left quadrant (ULQ), upper right quadrant (URQ), and lower central location (lower), all referenced to an electrode on the leg. Note that 3-cpm activity is seen more clearly in the EGG recordings than in the balloon recording. The first wave detected by the balloon recording was seen in the ULG and lower EGG recordings. It was not seen in the URQ EGG. Today EGG electrodes are placed in a location that is closer to the antrum. The second large wave detected by the balloon recording was associated with an EGG wave at the three EGG locations. (Reprinted with permission from Davis, Garafolo, and Kveim, 1959.)

Davis et al.[6] studied the effects of ingesting food on the EGG signal. They reported that the EGG showed very little activity when the stomach was empty, a controversial finding in light of the reports of so-called hunger contractions by Cannon and Washburn[7] and Carlson.[8] After recording the EGG from many fasted subjects both with and without a balloon in the stomach, Davis et al. contended that hunger contractions are rare and are usually stimulated by the introduction of a balloon into the stomach. Figure 1.5 shows the EGG of a fasted subject without a balloon (top tracing) and the EGG of the same subject recorded 10 minutes later with a balloon in the stomach (bottom three tracings). Note the increase in regular 3-cpm waves after the balloon is inflated in the stomach. The EGG signal is recorded with noninvasive techniques that do not interfere with normal ongoing activity of the stomach and provide novel insights into the understanding of gastric physiology.

Davis et al. (1957) developed the first procedure for hand scoring and quantification of EGG records. Records were divided into 30-second segments and quantified in terms of amplitude, frequency, and displacement (see Russell and Stern[9] for details). Amplitude was the favored measure in precomputer times because changes in amplitude were more obvious than the other measures. The amplitude of the EGG is still of interest today, but amplitude varies from subject to subject due to body mass, distance of electrodes from the stomach wall, and other factors. Amplitude also differs within the same subject from electrode site to electrode site because of varying distances from the stomach. Amplitude of the EGG signal also increases with contractions of the gastric muscle, but these changes may vary by type and intensity of contraction. Thus, an interpretation of EGG amplitude changes requires consideration of several factors.[10–12] *Displacement* was Davis' term for very slow changes in the EGG rhythm. It is now believed that some of what Davis called displacement was caused by inadequate techniques, such as electrode or amplifier drift, and some was ultra slow wave activity, such as less than 0.5 cycles per minute (cpm). We[13] have noted the presence of ultra slow wave activity in the EGG, as have others.[14]

The equipment used to record the EGG in 1960 was very crude by current standards. Appropriate silver/silver chloride electrodes were not commercially available. Experimenters constructed electrodes by cutting out square pieces of silver, soldering a wire to the back of each, and then electroplating the electrode, creating a silver/silver chloride

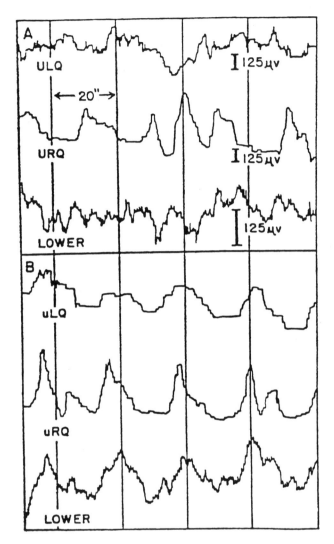

Figure 1.5. (A) Electrogastrogram (EGG) recordings from three locations in a fasted subject: upper left quadrant (ULQ), upper right quadrant (URQ), and a lower central location. Little 3-cpm activity is evident. (B) EGG activity from the same subject 10 minutes after the inflation of a balloon in the stomach. Note the clear 3-cpm EGG activity in response to inflation of the balloon. 20″ indicates 20 seconds. (Reprinted with permission from Davis, Garafolo, and Kveim, 1959.)

electrode to minimize polarization. DC amplifiers and strip-chart recorders were used with an external voltage to balance the offset potential between the active and reference electrodes. Automobile batteries were used as a power source for the amplifiers because there was too much alternating current electrical noise in commercially available direct current power supplies.

Two students working in Davis's laboratory conducted a noteworthy EGG study in the 1960s that was not published until a decade later. Stevens and Worrall[15] used cats to assess the validity of the EGG. Strain-gauge recordings from the serosal surface of the stomach and EGG recordings were obtained simultaneously. Frequencies recorded from the two sites were compared visually, and a very high correlation was found. However, what makes this study noteworthy is the fact that Stevens and Worrall used a fast paper speed in their polygraph and digitized strain-gauge and EGG signals by hand, once per second, and then performed what was perhaps the first Fourier analysis of the EGG.

In 1962, Sobakin, Smirnov, and Mishin[16] recorded the EGG in 164 patients and 61 healthy controls and reported that ulcers caused no change in the EGG but that pyloric stenosis produced a doubling of amplitude and that stomach cancer caused disruption of the normal 3-cpm rhythm. This was probably the first large-scale clinical use of the EGG.

Beginning in 1967, Martin and Murat and their colleagues in Tours, France, published numerous EGG studies[17] and an edited volume of gastric electrical recordings.[18] Their experiments included EGG validity studies in humans and animals, studies of the effects of stress and eating on EGG, and diagnostic studies using EGG recordings from patients with various diseases.

In 1968, Nelsen and Kohatsu[19] forced researchers to rethink the relationship of the EGG to contractions of the stomach. Up until that time, investigators assumed that the surface EGG recordings were related to contractions of the smooth muscle of the stomach. However, according to Nelsen and Kohatsu, the EGG reflected gastric slow wave activity, the electrical pacesetter potential activity of the stomach. They maintained that the EGG can be used to determine the frequency of contractions if and when they do occur, a circumstance that is distinct from the ongoing 3-cpm slow wave activity that is usually present in the stomach. They stressed that the EGG could not be used to detect the occurrence of gastric contractions.

Beginning in 1975, Duthie and his colleagues in Sheffield, England, published a number of studies[20,21] in which they examined the frequency of the EGG and made numerous advances in techniques for analysis of the EGG signal. In some of their studies, they compared the EGG with intragastric pressure recordings. Their conclusions were similar to those of Nelsen and Kohatsu. When contractions occurred, they occurred at the same frequency as the EGG. Although the EGG from most subjects showed 3 cpm almost continuously, contractions as recorded with intragastric pressure did not occur with such regularity. We now know that intragastric pressure recording instruments are not sensitive enough to record non–lumen-occluding contractions of the stomach or other low-amplitude contractile activity occurring in a particular part of the stomach.

During this same time, Andre Smout, Evert van der Schee, and their colleagues at the University of Rotterdam and Utrecht conducted several validation studies of the EGG and made major contributions in the area of signal analysis. In their landmark 1980 paper, "What Is Measured in Electrogastrography?"[22] they showed that the amplitude of the EGG increases when contractions occur. They also demonstrated the use of running spectral analysis (RSA), a technique for displaying EGG data in the frequency and time domain. RSA is used in many laboratories today and is described in detail in Chapter 5.

It was also about this same time, 1980, that Stern and Koch began their collaboration. One of the first studies they did involved the simultaneous recording of the EGG and fluoroscopy of the barium-filled stomach.[23] The correspondence between individual EGG waves and antral peristaltic contractions was observed repeatedly during simultaneous EGG-fluoroscopy recordings and is described in Chapter 3. Subsequently, these authors published a number of psychological and medical papers that focused on changes in EGG frequency during a variety of stressors, including motion and in patients with nausea and gastric neuromuscular disorders.

Clinical use of the EGG by gastroenterologists is increasing rapidly due to the ease, quality, and reliability of the recording methods for detecting normal gastric myoelectrical rhythms and gastric dysrhythmias. Increased knowledge about the relationship among gastric dysrhythmias, delayed gastric emptying, and nausea is evolving. Novel pharmaceutical agents and electrical pacing of the stomach are exciting new therapeutic areas requiring EGG recordings to diagnose dysrhythmias, develop rational approaches to therapy, and assess results of treatment. The recent increase in the use of the EGG by gastroenterologists has brought with it refinements in both hardware and software, including an ambulatory unit that has flown on Space Shuttle flights in an effort to learn more about the relationship of gastric electrical activity and space motion sickness.[24]

References

1. Alvarez WC: New methods of studying gastric peristalsis. *JAMA* 1922;22: 1281–1284.
2. Tumpeer IH, Blitzsten PW: Registration of peristalsis by the Einthoven galvonometer. *Am J Dis Child* 1926;21:454–455.
3. Tumpeer IH, Phillips B: Hyperperistaltic electrographic effects. *Am J Med Sci* 1932;184:831–836.
4. Stern RM, Stacher G: Recording the electrogastrogram from parts of the body surface distant from the stomach. *Psychophysiology* 1982;19:350.
5. Davis RC, Garafolo L, Gault FP: An exploration of abdominal potentials. *J Compar Physiol Psychol* 1957;50:519–523.
6. Davis RC, Garafolo L, Kveim K: Conditions associated with gastrointestinal activity. *J Compar Physiol Psychol* 1959;52:466–475.
7. Cannon WB, Washburn AL: An explanation of hunger. *Am J Physiol* 1912;29:441–454.
8. Carlson AJ: The relation between the contractions of the empty stomach and the sensation of hunger. *Am J Physiol* 1912;31:175–192.
9. Russell RW, Stern RM: Gastric motility: the electrogastrogram. In: Venables PH, Martin I, eds. *A Manual of Psychophysiological Methods.* Amsterdam: North-Holland Publishing Co;1967:219–243.
10. Mintchev MP, Kingma YJ, Bowes KL: Accuracy of cutaneous recordings of gastric electrical activity. *Gastroenterology* 1993;104:1273–1280.
11. Mintchev MP, Bowes KL: Extracting quantitative information from digital electrogastrogrms. *Med Biolog Eng Comput* 1996;34:244–248.
12. Dubois A, Mizrahi M: Electrogastrography, gastric emptying, and gastric motility. In: Chen JZ, McCallum RW, eds. *Electrogastrography, Principles and Applications.* New York: Raven Press;1994:247–256.
13. Stern RM, Koch KL, Stewart WR, et al: Spectral analysis of tachygastria recorded during motion sickness. *Gastroenterologist* 1987;92:92–97.
14. Holzl R, Loffler K, Muller GM: On conjoint gastrography or what the surface gastrograms show. In: Stern RM, Koch KL, eds. *Electrogastrography.* New York: Praeger;1985:89–115.
15. Stevens JK, Worrall N: External recording of gastric activity: the electrogastrogram. *Physiol Psychol* 1974;2:175–180.
16. Sobakin MA, Smirnov IP, Mishin LN: Electrogastrography. *IRE Trans Biomed Electr* 1962;9:129–132.

17. Martin A, Thouvenot J, Touron P: Periodic changes in abdominal cutaneous potentials in relation to digestive activity. *C R Soc Biol* (Paris) 1967;161:2595–2600.

18. Murat J, Dobrev J, Vaur JL, et al, eds.: *Enregistrements Clectriaues de la motricite digestive: applications medico-chirurgicales.* [Electrical recordings of digestive motility: Medical-surgical applications.] Tours, France: University of Tours, 1975.

19. Nelsen TS, Kohatsu S: Clinical electrogastrography and its relationship to gastric surgery. *Am J Surg* 1968;116:215–222.

20. Brown BH, Smallwood R, Duthie HL, et al: Intestinal smooth muscle electrical potentials recorded from surface electrodes. *Med Biol Eng* 1975;11:97–103.

21. Smallwood RH: Analysis of gastric electrical signals from surface electrodes using phase-lock techniques. Part 2, C system performance with gastric signals. *Med Biol Eng Comput* 1978;16:513–518.

22. Smout AJPM, van der Schee EJ, Grashuis JL: What is measured in electrogastrography? *Dig Dis Sci* 1980;25:179–187.

23. Koch KL, Stewart WR, Stern RM: The relationship between the cutaneously recorded electrogastrogram and antral contractions in man. In: Stern RM, Koch KL, eds. *Electrogastrography: Methodology, Validation and Applications.* New York: Praeger Publishers, 1985;116–131.

24. Harm DL, Sandoz GR, Stern RM: Changes in gastric myoelectrical activity during space flight. *Dig Dis Sci* 2002;47:1737–1745.

2

Properties of Electrical Rhythmicity in the Stomach

Kenton M. Sanders, Tamas Ördög,
Sang Don Koh, and Sean M. Ward

G astric peristaltic contractions are the basis for emptying of solids from the stomach.[1] These events begin in the mid to high corpus region, develop into a ring around the stomach, and spread down the length of the stomach to the pylorus. The pressure wave resulting from gastric peristalsis pushes the contents of the stomach toward the pyloric sphincter, but a nearly simultaneous contraction of the ring of muscle in the pyloric canal and the terminal antrum ultimately forces much of the food in the retrograde direction, toward the body of the stomach. Sheer forces that develop as a result of this forceful retropulsion cause mechanical disruption of solid particles. Repetitive peristaltic contractions (e.g., in the human these events occur about 3 times per minute), over a period of time, reduces ingested foods to small particles. The action of gastric peristalsis in the distal stomach facilitates emptying and the reduced particle diameter aides in chemical digestion of foods in the small intestine. Pathophysiological conditions that disrupt or disorganize gastric peristalsis can impair or delay normal gastric emptying.

Gastric peristaltic contractions result from depolarization of the plasma membranes of smooth muscle cells. For many years it has been known that gastric muscles display periodic (or rhythmic) electrical activity in which membrane potential oscillates between negative potentials and more depolarized levels. The oscillations in membrane potential are known as electrical slow waves (see Color Figs. 2.1 and 2.2 in separate color insert). Slow waves are generated within the tunica muscularis of the proximal corpus along the greater curvature of the stomach, and these events spread around the circumference and down the stomach to the pylorus. A greater velocity of propagation around the stomach than down the stomach causes development of a ring of excitation, and this is the electrical basis underlying gastric peristaltic contractions.

Studies have shown that electrical slow waves are generated by specialized pacemaker cells, known as interstitial cells of Cajal (ICCs). The main pacemaker ICCs in the stomach form a dense network of electrically coupled cells between the circular and longitudinal muscle layers of the corpus and antrum. These cells generate and actively propagate slow waves throughout the musculature of the distal stomach. Both circular and longitudinal smooth muscle cells are electrically coupled to the network of ICCs, and electrical slow waves conduct to the smooth muscle cells via these connections. Smooth muscle cells do not possess the means to generate or actively propagate slow waves, but the depolarization caused by slow waves causes activation of a variety of voltage-dependent ion channels in the smooth muscle cell membrane. For example, gastric smooth muscle cells express voltage-dependent Ca^{2+} channels that are activated over the voltage range of slow waves. Thus, during the slow wave cycle, opening of Ca^{2+} channels causes influx of Ca^{2+} into gastric smooth muscle cells, and this initiates contraction. Enteric motor nerves "condition" the response of the musculature to slow wave activity. Release of inhibitory neurotransmitters hyperpolarizes postjunctional membrane potential and tends to decrease the probability of Ca^{2+} channel openings and reduce contractile responses. Release of excitatory neurotransmitter increases coupling between slow wave depolarization and Ca^{2+} channel activation and increases the force of contraction (see Color Fig. 2.1 in separate color insert).

Although the dominant pacemaker of the stomach is situated in the corpus, each region of the stomach below this site possesses pacemaker capability. This is because the ICC network is extensive and infiltrates most of the musculature of the corpus and antrum. Each region, therefore, is capable of producing (or regenerating) slow

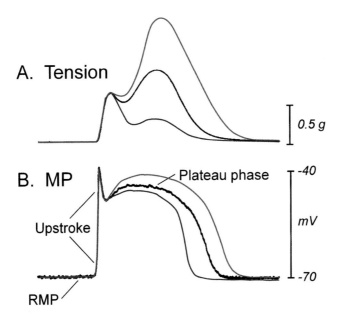

A. Tension

0.5 g

B. MP

Plateau phase

-40

Upstroke

mV

-70

RMP

Color Figure 2.1. Gastric slow waves and contractile responses. (*A and B*) Membrane potential (MP) and a typical slow wave event (*B*) with the associated contractile response (*A*) from the canine antral circular muscle (black traces). Excitatory stimuli (red traces) and inhibitory stimuli (blue) alter the wave forms of the slow waves and the contractile responses coupled to the slow wave. These traces are superimposed, idealized traces. Small changes in the plateau amplitude translate into significant changes in the amplitude of the contractile response. RMP, resting membrane potential.

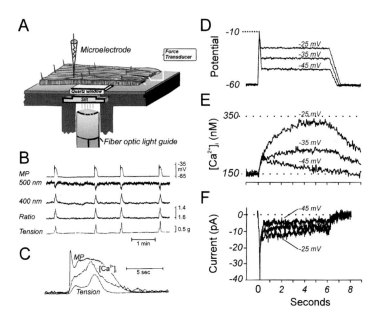

Color Figure 2.2. Coupling between slow waves, Ca^{2+}, and contraction. (*A*) shows apparatus to measure electrical activity and changes in intracellular Ca^{2+} and contractile responses. Muscle is pinned to the base of a recording chamber with a quartz window. A slit allows excitation light to excite the dye loaded in the tissue. A microelectrode is used to impale cells close to the site of optical recording, and a force transducer records contractions of a small region of muscle from the same area. (*B*) Simultaneous recordings of membrane potential (MP), optical signals (indo-1–loaded smooth muscle tissue), and tension. The optical signals are emissions at 400 and 500 nm in response to excitation with 340-nm light. These signals were ratioed (ratio traces) to give an indication of changes in intracellular Ca^{2+}. Tension shows the contractile response. (C) Superposition of one of the slow waves (MP), Ca^{2+}, and contractile responses. Note that depolarization precedes the Ca^{2+} transient, and tension follows the rise in intracellular Ca^{2+}. (These data are redrawn from Ozaki et al., 1991.) (D–F) Voltage-clamp and simultaneous membrane currents and changes in intracellular Ca^{2+} in an isolated canine antral myocyte. The voltage clamp was programmed to produce a command potential to simulate a gastric slow wave (*D*). The plateaus phase of the command potential were adjusted (−45 to −25) to simulate a normal slow wave (−35 mV) and a slow wave during excitatory (−25 mV) or inhibitory (−45 mV) influences. Note the small effect on inward currents elicited (*F*), and the rather dramatic effects on intracellular Ca^{2+} (*E*) during voltage-clamp steps over this range. (Data are reproduced from Vogalis et al., 1991.)

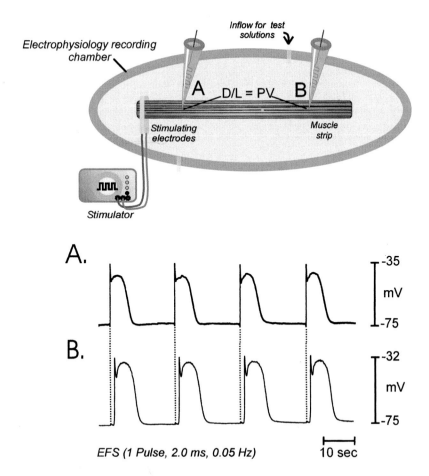

Color Figure 2.4. Active propagation of gastric slow waves. (*Top*) Set-up and conditions to measure propagation from a strip of smooth muscle. Gastric strips were placed in a chamber with stimulating electrodes at one end. Two microelectrodes were used to make simultaneous recordings from cells at either end of the strip. Distance was measured between the tips of the microelectrodes. Distance (D) divided by latency (L) of arrival of the slow waves at the two electrodes equals the propagation velocity (PV). Traces A and B show records of evoked slow waves recorded at electrodes A and B. Dotted lines denote the latency between the stimulus and the arrival of the slow wave at electrode B. Note that the waveforms of the events recorded at the two sites. This demonstrates that propagation is active (i.e., due to a regenerative mechanism).

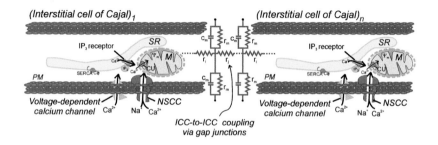

Color Figure 2.6. Mechanism of electrical pacemaking in gastrointestinal muscles. Pacemaker currents arise from subcellular compartments composed a region of plasma membrane (PM) that is associated with sarcoplasmic reticulum (SR) and mitochondria (M). Each region of an ICC with this structural arrangement might be considered a pacemaker unit. Two of these pacemaker units are depicted in the figure. Release of Ca^{2+} via IP_3 receptors triggers the pacemaker event. The cell in which this first occurs is considered the primary pacemaker (ICC_1). Ca^{2+} release from IP_3 receptors triggers uptake of Ca^{2+} into mitochondria down its electrochemical gradient (Ψ_m). The decrease in local Ca^{2+} resulting from mitochondrial uptake activates a Ca^{2+}-inhibited nonselective cation conductance (NSCC) in the plasma membrane. Reuptake of Ca^{2+} by the SERCA pump resets this mechanism. The rate at which the IP_3 release event occurs in a given pacemaker unit may depend on leak of Ca^{2+} through a dihydropyridine-resistant Ca^{2+} conductance or another undetermined conductance. The inward current entering the ICC_1 via the NSCC causes depolarization of this cell and neighboring cells through the gap junctions that connect ICCs into a network. The depolarization of neighboring cells is dependent on the cable properties of the ICC network, including elements such as membrane capacitance (c_m), membrane resistance (r_m), internal cytoplasmic resistance (c_i), and junctional resistance (r_j). Depolarization initiates Ca^{2+} entry in coupled cells via activation of voltage-dependent Ca^{2+} channels. Although ICC express L-type Ca^{2+} channels, this conductance does not appear to be necessary for pacemaker propagation. A voltage-dependent, dihydropyridine-resistant Ca^{2+} conductance is also present in ICCs, and this appears to be sufficient to sustain propagation. Ca^{2+} entry near secondary pacemaker units (ICC_n) enhances the probability of IP_3 receptor-operated Ca^{2+} release and initiates regeneration of the pacemaker current. This is hypothesized to be the entraining signal that facilitates active propagation of slow waves through networks of ICC

wave activity. The orderly generation and propagation of slow waves in the stomach depends on a gradient in the intrinsic frequency at which slow waves are generated. For example, the frequency of slow waves in the proximal corpus is about 3 per minute in the human, but only about 1 per minute in the mid antrum. The corpus pacemaker is "dominant," not because it is the sole pacemaker region in the stomach but because it generates slow waves at the greatest frequency. The corpus pacemaker dominates because there is time for slow waves generated in this region to propagate and initiate slow waves at more distal sites before these sites can generate their own event. Motility disorders can result when there is a breakdown in the gastric frequency gradient, because the time required for slow wave propagation may not be sufficient for the corpus pacemaker to entrain distal pacemakers. In such cases, normal spread of peristaltic contractions from corpus to pylorus is inhibited. Dysrhythmias can result either from acceleration of the antral pacemaker frequency, deceleration of the corpus pacemaker, development of ectopic (abnormally high frequency) pacemakers, or defects in the propagation pathway (e.g., disruptions in the continuity of the ICC network). This chapter discusses the properties of the gastric electrical slow waves, the slow wave frequency gradient, characteristics of gastric slow wave propagation, pacemaker currents generated by ICCs, the mechanism of pacemaker activity, regulation of pacemaker frequency, and the likely basis of some gastric dysrhythmias. Based on the physiology (and physics!) of gastric electrophysiology, we also discuss some of the problems encountered by clinicians attempting to diagnose problems related to gastric dysrhythmias.

Properties of Gastric Electrical Slow Waves

In intact pieces of gastric muscle, the membrane potentials of corpus and antral smooth muscle cells are not constant. Membrane potential oscillates between about -60 to $-75\,\text{mV}$ and -20 to $-40\,\text{mV}$. The most negative potential reached during this cycle is typically referred to as the *resting membrane potential*, and the term is applicable because at these potentials, the opening of Ca^{2+} channels is infrequent, Ca^{2+} entry is minimal, and the muscle cells tend to be relaxed. Electrical slow waves in gastric muscles are generated by a specialized population of cells between the circular and longitudinal

muscle layers known as ICCs. This idea is based on the temporal relationship between slow waves recorded from ICCs and smooth muscle cells in small strips of gastric muscle[2] and the fact that gastric
muscles lacking ICCs do not display slow wave activity.[3] Gastric slow
waves have distinctive waveforms consisting of a relatively rapid upstroke depolarization, followed by partial repolarization, and a
plateau potential that can last for several seconds (see Color Fig. 2.1
in separate color insert). In the distal stomach, there often are a series
of more rapid oscillations superimposed on the plateau phase of the
slow waves. In the gastric literature, these events are often referred to
as "spike potentials." There often is a stable resting potential between
slow waves, and the onset of the slow wave is characterized by expo-
nential development of depolarization, indicating propagation of
these events from another region of the tissue.

   Although slow waves can be recorded from essentially every
smooth muscle cell in the distal stomach, these events are not generated or regenerated by smooth muscle cells. Studies of isolated smooth
muscle cells have shown that the slow wave mechanism is absent from
these cells. Thus, slow waves are conducted to the musculature from another source. As discussed later, the ICCs of the myenteric region (i.e.,
area between circular and longitudinal muscle layer) are the primary
pacemakers in the stomach and the source of slow waves. Electrical connections between ICCs and smooth muscle cells allow passive conduction of slow waves to the muscle cells. Depolarization of the muscle
from the spread of slow waves activates voltage-dependent Ca^{2+} channels and entry of Ca^{2+}. Entry of Ca^{2+} is primarily due to activation of
"L-type" or dihydropyridine-sensitive Ca^{2+} channels. Thus, coupling between slow wave activity, Ca^{2+} entry, and contraction can be reduced or
blocked by Ca^{2+} channel antagonists, such as nifedipine or diltiazem.

   During slow waves, the amplitude of depolarization is such that
openings of individual L-type Ca^{2+} channels are relatively brief.
However, the duration of slow waves is such that the summated Ca^{2+}
entry through thousands of channels opening occasionally over several seconds results in net Ca^{2+} gain by cells. The increase in intracellular Ca^{2+} is sufficient to initiate a contractile response. The
minimum level of Ca^{2+} entry that couples to detectable contractions
has been referred to as the *mechanical threshold.*[4] Direct measurements of membrane potential, intracellular Ca^{2+}, and contractile
responses have clearly described the relationship and timing between these events[5] (see Color Fig. 2.2A–C in separate color insert).

This basic feature of excitation–contraction coupling can also be demonstrated in isolated smooth muscle cells[6] (see Color Fig. 2.2D–F in separate color insert). When these cells are held under voltage-clamp conditions and then depolarized with pulses that mimic the waveform of gastric slow waves, Ca^{2+} currents are activated, and this causes net increases in intracellular Ca^{2+}.

The relatively low level of Ca^{2+} channel activation during spontaneous slow wave activity provides a large dynamic range over which coupling between slow waves and contractions can be regulated. The steepness of the relationship between voltage and contraction[4] predicts that relatively small increases in the amplitude of slow waves can greatly increase Ca^{2+} entry and contractile responses. A variety of biogenic agonists, such as excitatory neurotransmitters, hormones, and paracrine substances, enhance the amplitudes of slow waves and increase the force of contractions (see Color Fig. 2.1 in separate color insert). This is the mechanism for conversion of weak contractions during fasting to very large, almost occlusive, contractions of the gastric musculature in the late postprandial period. Charles Code referred to these as type I and type II gastric contractions.[7]

The Slow Wave Frequency Gradient

ICCs generate the pacemaker currents responsible for slow waves, and extensive histological examinations of the stomachs of laboratory animals have shown that ICCs are extensively distributed in the pacemaker regions of the corpus and antrum of mammalian stomachs[8] (Fig. 2.3A–B). This is likely to be the basis for the observation that virtually every part of the distal stomach is spontaneously active.[9] Small strips of muscle dissected from areas from the orad corpus to the pylorus display spontaneous slow wave activity. A fundamental feature of the stomach that emerges from such recordings is that muscles from the corpus consistently generate slow waves at higher frequencies than muscles of the antrum. Thus, a frequency gradient exists where the intrinsic frequency of proximal muscle pacemakers is greater than the frequency of distal pacemakers. For example, in the canine stomach, the frequency in the orad corpus averaged 3.7 cycles per minute (cpm), and in the distal antrum, 0.7 cpm.[9] The frequency gradient is an extremely important property of gastric pacemakers, and breakdown (or reorganization) of this frequency gradient can have profound

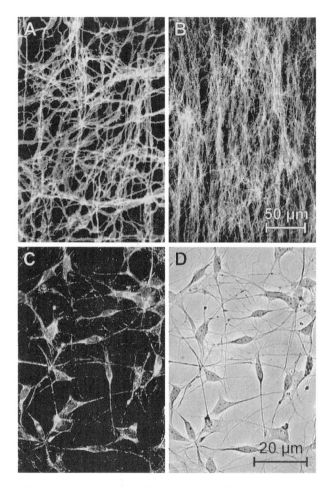

Figure 2.3. ICC networks in situ and in culture. ICCs (stained with an antibody for Kit receptors) are arranged into inconnected networks in the corpus (*A*) and antrum (*B*). The images were obtained with confocal microscopy and represent the cells in the myenteric regions between the circular and longitudinal muscle layers. These are the pacemaker ICCs in the stomach. *C* (Kit immunofluorescence) and *D* (phase contrast) show the same population of ICCs from the antrum in cell culture conditions. The cells form similar networks as occur in situ and retain the rhythmic phenotype of cells in situ.

18

effects on the performance of the stomach. Therefore, it is significant that this fundamental feature of gastric motility is encoded in the pacemaker mechanism of the ICCs residing in the different parts of the stomach.[8] ICCs from the corpus generate pacemaker currents at higher frequencies than antral ICCs. Thus, alterations in the intrinsic frequency of the ICCs in any region of the stomach could disrupt the gastric frequency gradient, giving rise to gastric arrhythmias and delayed emptying (see later). Better understanding of the cellular mechanisms that set the pacemaker frequencies of ICCs may lead to the development of specific treatments for different forms of dysrhythmias.

Characteristics of Slow Wave Propagation

For gastric peristalsis to spread as a mechanical wave, gastric slow waves must propagate through the tens of cm^3 of the gastric musculature. Because smooth muscle cells lack the mechanism of slow wave generation, active propagation must occur through ICC networks. The most important ICC network for slow wave generation and propagation lies in the myenteric region between the circular and longitudinal muscle layers of the corpus and antrum (IC-MY). The mechanism of slow wave propagation is not entirely understood at the present time. Measurements of propagation rates in the canine stomach have given values of 23 mm/sec in the long axis of the circular muscle fibers and 11 mm/sec in the long axis of the stomach.[10] These values are consistent with an electrical mechanism, although propagation rates in the stomach are slow in comparison to nerves and skeletal and cardiac muscles. Slow waves propagate with relatively little change in waveform over many centimeters of gastric tissue (i.e., propagation occurs without significant decrement; see Color Fig. 2.4 in separate color insert). Thus, an active mechanism exists in which slow waves are regenerated as they spread from cell to cell. The regeneration mechanism must reside within the ICC network, because gastric muscles that have lost ICCs are not capable of regenerating slow waves.[3,8,11] Slow waves conduct into smooth muscle cells but are not actively propagated by these cells. Slow waves decay in amplitude and disappear within a few millimeters in a region of gastric muscle devoid of ICCs. Thus, patients with even partial loss of ICC networks may experience loss of slow waves in regions lacking ICCs. This may leave areas of the stomach uncontrolled by slow wave activity and therefore unable to participate in gastric peristaltic contractions.

The myenteric ICC networks (IC-MYs) lies in a plane between the circular and longitudinal muscle layers. IC-MYs may be sufficient for propagation of slow waves in small animals with thin muscle layers. Conduction of slow waves through a thin layer of muscle does not result in sufficient attenuation of the slow wave to affect function. In humans and other mammals, however, with muscle layers many millimeters in thickness, slow waves must also be regenerated through the depth of the muscle layers. Measurements of propagation velocity through the circular muscle layer (i.e., from the myenteric border to the submucosal border) have shown that slow waves propagate at 10 mm/sec.[10] It has been proposed that a specialized propagation network of ICCs, for example, the septal ICCs that line the muscle bundles of the circular muscle layer, may be used for this function.[12]

Pacemaker Currents Generated by Interstitial Cells of Cajal

It is now possible to isolate and culture ICCs (see Color Fig. 2.4 in separate color insert), and studies of these cells have revealed much about the slow wave pacemaker mechanism. ICCs in primary culture retain their rhythmic phenotype for several days. With proper culturing techniques, it is possible to obtain small clusters of ICCs, and the ICCs within these clusters form electrical connections with each other. Thus, it is possible to perform voltage-clamp experiments to investigate the properties of the pacemaker currents that underlie slow waves.

ICCs from the murine gastric antrum display regular inward currents at an average of 1 cycle per minute[13] (Fig. 2.5). These events consist of a rapid phase and a plateau current lasting several seconds. In current-clamp mode, it can be seen that the spontaneous inward currents elicit slow wave–like depolarizations in ICCs. These events were not blocked by dihydropyridines, which is characteristic of slow waves recorded from intact strips of gastric muscle. Studies have suggested that the intracellular pacemaker mechanism and membrane ionic channels responsible for producing pacemaker currents are not voltage dependent.

Although not thoroughly investigated at the present time, the pacemaker currents of the stomach appear to be similar, although slower in frequency, to the pacemaker currents of small intestinal ICCs.

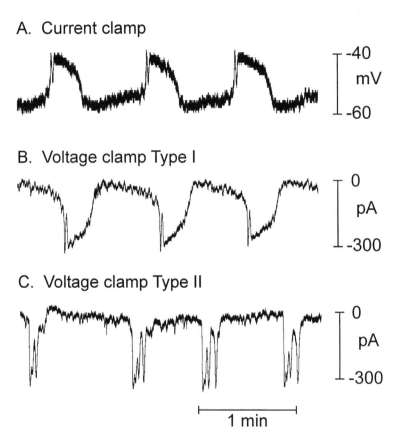

Figure 2.5. Pacemaker activity of gastric interstitial cells of Cajal (ICCs). ICCs isolated from antral tissues were cultured for 1 to 3 days. (*A*) The cells were spontaneously active, producing events similar to the slow waves recorded in situ. (*B and C*) show pacemaker currents recorded under voltage clamp conditions. We observed two types of current patterns; *B* shows type 1 currents consisting of a sharp inward current followed by a plateau phase (same cell as in *A*). (*C*) Currents with multiple peaks. This type of current pattern is reminiscent of the activity recorded from tissues in the terminal antrum or pylorus.

A nonselective cation conductance generates the pacemaker current in ICCs.[14] This is an unusual current because it is inhibited by intracellular Ca^{2+}, and the openings of the channels are regulated by binding of Ca^{2+}/calmodulin. At high intracellular Ca^{2+}, the conductance is inactive, but when Ca^{2+} is lowered or cells are treated with calmodulin inhibitors, a significant enhancement in pacemaker currents occurs or, in extreme cases, a tonic inward current is activated.

Mechanism of Pacemaker Activity

Two fundamental questions arise from the studies of the properties of the pacemaker current: (1) How are the pacemaker channels activated in a rhythmic manner? (2) How do slow waves propagate through ICCs? Studies of cultured ICCs have produced novel concepts for the mechanism of pacemaker activity in gastrointestinal smooth muscles. Pacemaker activity begins when Ca^{2+} is released from inositol trisphosphate (IP_3) receptor–operated stores in the sarcoplasmic reticulum of ICCs.[15,16] A significant study demonstrating the importance of this step was performed in mice genetically lacking IP_3 type 1 receptors. Gastric muscles of these animals did not have the ability to generate electrical slow waves.[17] There are many sites where IP_3-dependent Ca^{2+} release can occur in networks of ICCs, but the site where this occurs first (and is reinforced by other events) is the primary pacemaker cell for a given cycle. Leak of Ca^{2+} through membrane conductances such as cation channels or dihydropyridine-resistant Ca^{2+} channels may enhance the rate at which the primary pacemaker event occurs, and it has been known for many years that reducing extracellular Ca^{2+} slows pacemaker frequency. IP_3 receptors lie in close proximity to mitochondria, and release of Ca^{2+} from IP_3 receptors triggers Ca^{2+} uptake by mitochondria via a Ca^{2+}-dependent transporter (CU). The sarcoplasmic reticulum–mitochondria complexes lie close to the plasma membrane, and mitochondrial Ca^{2+} uptake transiently reduces Ca^{2+} activity in the space close to the plasma membrane. It is the reduction of Ca^{2+} in this space that activates the Ca^{2+}-inhibited, nonselective cation conductance (I_{NSCC}) described earlier (see section on pacemaker currents generated by ICCs). Ultimately, this process also depends on reuptake of Ca^{2+} into the IP_3 receptor–operated stores by Ca^{2+}-ATPases (SERCA pumps) in the sarcoplasmic reticulum to reset the mechanism. This model is illustrated in Color Figure 2.6 (in separate color insert).

It is interesting to note that the stochastic nature of this pacemaker mechanism suggests that no single ICC is always the primary pacemaker in a network of ICCs. In studies where activity was mapped in gastric muscles, the site of origin of pacemaker events shifted from place to place as a function of time.[18] This happens in relatively small clusters of ICCs or in small bits of tissue because the frequency of pacemaker activity in one cell is not significantly different than the frequency of another. Large-scale shifting of the primary pacemaker does not normally happen on a macroscale in the whole stomach (e.g., proximal to distal) because the frequency of corpus pacemaking is consistently greater than the antral pacemaker frequency. Thus, the corpus always dominates in stomach when the normal proximal-to-distal frequency gradient exists. The anatomical basis for entrainment is the connections between pacemaker ICCs, as demonstrated in cultures of gastric ICCs, where faster, corpus ICCs couple with slower, antral ICCs and entrain the pacemaker activity of the antral ICCs.[8]

Propagation of electrical activity in excitable cells or networks of excitable cells typically uses the voltage-dependent properties of the channels responsible for active events to regenerate activity over distance. From nerves to cardiac muscles, there are significant similarities in propagation mechanisms. Depolarization of one cell or region of membrane activates voltage-dependent conductances ahead of the site of activity and regenerates the event. The pacemaker current in ICCs does not manifest voltage-dependent properties, but the rate of propagation of slow waves in intact tissues dictates that an electrical mechanism must be integrated with the pacemaker mechanism to achieve active propagation (see section on characteristics of slow wave propagation). Another requirement is that the electrical mechanism, in most cases, involved in propagation is not dependent on dihydropyridine-sensitive Ca^{2+} channels. ICCs express voltage-dependent, dihydropyridine-resistant Ca^{2+} channels,[19] and these channels may participate in the mechanism of active propagation via the following model. The inward current generated by activation of the pacemaker conductance in the primary pacemaker depolarizes adjacent ICCs via current spread through the gap junctions that couple these cells into a network. The magnitude and region influenced by the depolarization depend on the cable properties of the ICC network. Depolarization of neighboring ICC activates voltage-dependent Ca^{2+} channels, and Ca^{2+} entry in the space near IP_3

receptors promotes (i.e., phase advances) Ca^{2+} release and reactivation of the pacemaker mechanism. This mechanism is illustrated in Color Figure 2.6 in separate color insert.

The rate of propagation in ICC networks is considerably slower than propagation in many excitable cells. Ca^{2+} entry and buildup may be the delaying factor that slows down propagation of slow waves. Other ideas for propagation include voltage-dependent regulation of IP_3 production where depolarization from the primary pacemaker causes enhanced production of IP_3 in coupled ICCs.[20] Raising IP_3 levels would also tend to set off the pacemaker mechanism, so this hypothesis should be given serious consideration. It is also possible that there is a link between voltage-dependent Ca^{2+} entry and IP_3 production. Some phospholipase C (PLC) enzymes, which synthesize IP_3, are regulated by Ca^{2+}. Thus, Ca^{2+} entry could stimulate PLC activity ahead of a propagating slow wave, and induce regeneration by enhancing production of IP_3. Testing of this mechanism requires the use of a sensitive bioprobe or fluorescent indicator that can sense small changes in IP_3 concentration.

Regulation of Pacemaker Frequency

Regulation of pacemaker frequency is critical in gastric muscles. As discussed earlier, proper organization of electrical activity in the stomach requires the maintenance of a frequency gradient from the proximal to the distal stomach. The regulation of frequency has been studied in cultured gastric ICCs, and several predictions can now be made about

$\longrightarrow$

Figure 2.7. Regulation of pacemaker frequency in antral interstitial cells of Cajal (ICCs). (*A*) Effects of forskolin (FSK) on pacemaker currents. FSK, which stimulates the production of cAMP, greatly decreases the frequency of pacemaker currents. Drugs that mimic cAMP have the same effect. (*B*) Muscarinic stimulation of murine antral muscles increases slow wave frequency and induces tonic depolarization. (*C*) Positive chronotropic effects of ACh are manifest on ICC. Pacemaker currents are increased in frequency, and this effect is superimposed on a small increase in tonic inward current. (*D*) Regulation of slow wave frequency by an EP_3 agonist, ONO-AE-248. First trace shows control slow wave activity, middle trace shows effects of ONO-AE-248, and third trace shows restoration of control conditions after washout of ONO-AE-248. (*E*) Effects of another EP_3 agonist, GR 63799X, on pacemaker current frequency in antral ICC. Note the profound chronotropic effect of this compound.

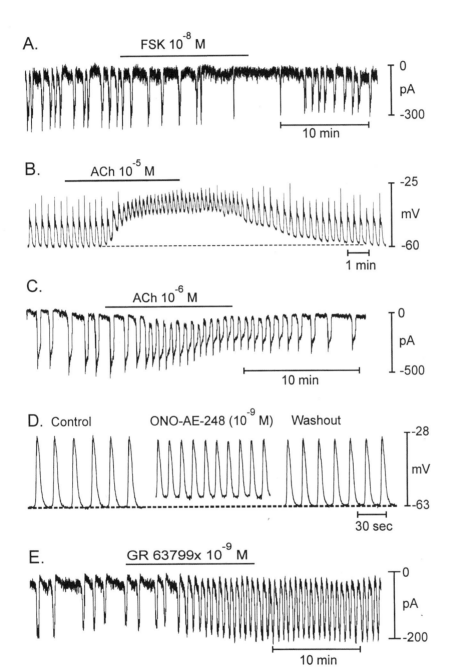

A. FSK 10^{-8} M

0
pA
−300

|— 10 min —|

B. ACh 10^{-5} M

−25
mV
−60

|— 1 min —|

C. ACh 10^{-6} M

0
pA
−500

|— 10 min —|

D. Control ONO-AE-248 (10^{-9} M) Washout

−28
mV
−63

|— 30 sec —|

E. GR 63799x 10^{-9} M

0
pA
−200

|— 10 min —|

25

how various drugs and biogenic agonists will affect slow wave frequency. Forskolin, a drug that activates adenyl cyclase in cells, slows and can even stop pacemaker currents in ICCs[13] (Fig. 2-7A). Similarly, membrane-permeable analogues of cyclic adenosine monophosphate (cAMP) slowed pacemaker frequency. Thus, compounds coupled to the production of cAMP in gastric ICCs should have negative chronotropic effects on pacemaker activity. This hypothesis has been verified in intact gastric muscles.[21,22] Negative chronotropic effects were also elicited by drugs that stimulate production of cyclic guanosine monophosphate (cGMP) or mimic cGMP. Two of the major inhibitory neurotransmitters—vasoactive intestinal polypeptide (VIP) and nitric oxide (NO)—and several gastrointestinal hormones are linked to cyclic nucleotide production. Thus, the release of these compounds and expression of receptors for these compounds by ICC may be linked to negative chronotropic effects in gastric ICCs, in the absence of additional coupling of the receptors to other mechanisms.

A more interesting side of regulation, however, is the ability of some compounds to greatly accelerate pacemaker activity. This is particularly important in the antral region of the stomach, because increasing antral frequency can result in a breakdown in the gastric frequency gradient and blockade of gastric peristalsis. It has been known that cholinergic stimulation increases slow wave frequency, and similar regulation occurs in the murine stomach (Fig. 2.7B). ICCs from the murine antrum are also stimulated by cholinergic agonists, and pacemaker frequency is greatly increased in these cells by acetylcholine and carbachol[23] (Fig. 2.7C). This occurs via M_3 receptors, as a selective M_3 antagonist blocked the chronotropic effect with high potency. Other tests suggested that the major coupling between M_3 receptors and the chronotropic response in ICCs is the production of IP_3. An increase in pacemaker frequency with elevated IP_3 is consistent with the model for slow wave generation, because the first step in that mechanism is release of Ca^{2+} from IP_3 receptor-operated stores (see section on mechanism of pacemaker activity). Enhancing IP_3 production and local concentration should accelerate openings of IP_3 receptors and phase advance the generation of slow waves.

Studies of tachygastria in humans and animal models have identified prostaglandin E_2 (PGE_2) as a primary agonist that induces positive chronotropic effects.[24,25] We verified that slow wave frequency in murine antral muscles is enhanced by PGE_2.[13] Exposure of cultured ICCs to

PGE_2, however, greatly decreased pacemaker frequency. The effects of PGE_2 are mediated by several isoforms of PGE_2 receptors (EP_1 to EP_4). It was found that EP_2 and EP_4 selective agonists reduced slow wave frequency in tissues and pacemaker frequency in ICC. These receptors are coupled to both adenylyl cyclase and production of cAMP. Thus, slowing of frequency with these compounds is consistent with the actions of cAMP. Several EP_3 receptor agonists stimulated slow wave frequency in tissues and ICCs (see Fig. 2.7D–E). Thus, the EP_3 isoform appears to couple PGE_2 to positive chonotropic effects. The switch in the dominant response of cultured ICCs to PGE_2 from a positive chonotropic effect to inhibition of pacemaker frequency is likely to be due to the balance between EP_2/EP_4 receptors and EP_3 receptors in these cells. At present, we are unsure of the second messenger(s) responsible for the positive chonotropic effects of EP_3 receptors, but these receptors have been linked to inhibition of cAMP production and enhanced production of IP_3. Both of these pathways tend to enhance slow wave frequency. These findings suggest that an EP_3 antagonist could be useful in treating gastric arrhythmias associated with an overabundance of PGE_2. The data also suggest the hypothesis that in some of the patients who have gastric tachygastrias, either an increase in prostaglandins or an imbalance in prostaglandin receptor expression (i.e., upregulation of EP_3 receptors) could account for symptoms.

Basis of Some Gastric Dysrhythmias

Gastric dysrhythmias may accompany a wide variety of conditions, such as diabetic and idiopathic gastroparesis, functional dyspepsia, nausea during pregnancy, chronic mesenteric ischemia, chronic intestinal obstruction, abdominal malignancies, anorexia nervosa, motion sickness, chronic renal failure, and unexplained nausea and vomiting.[26] A host of neural and humoral factors (including those discussed in the previous section) have been proposed to elicit aberrant patterns of gastric myoelectrical activity in these conditions. Studies of the pacemaker mechanism in ICCs and integration of slow wave activity in intact muscles and stomachs have provided an ability to understand or predict the cause(s) of some gastric arrhythmias. As we more thoroughly understand how various stimuli affect the pacemaker mechanism, it may be possible to develop criteria for grouping arrhythmias on the basis of mechanism rather than by frequency.

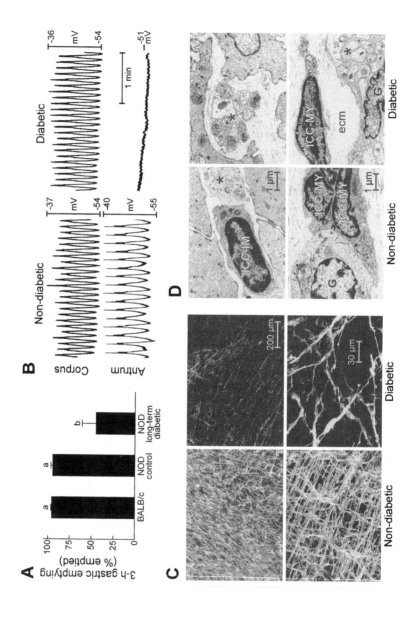

A

3-h gastric emptying (% emptied)

B

Non-diabetic   Diabetic

Corpus

Antrum

1 min

C

Non-diabetic   Diabetic

200 μm

30 μm

D

Non-diabetic   Diabetic

ICC-IM

ICC-MY
ICC-MY

ICC-MY

ecm

G

G

1 μm

1 μm

Figure 2.8. Effects of diabetes mellitus on gastric emptying of solids (*A*), electrical slow wave activity (*B*), and ICCs (*C, D*) in NOD mice. (*A*) Gastric emptying of solid food after 3 hours in normal BALB/c, control NOD, and long-term diabetic (>1.5 months) NOD mice. Data are expressed as percent emptying of solids. Gastric emptying in long-term diabetic mice was significantly reduced relative to control groups. (*B*) Representative recordings of spontaneous activity in the corpus and antrum of normal (left) and diabetic (right) NOD mice. Rhythmic slow waves were recorded throughout the corpus and antrum in control animals. In diabetic animals, most of the cells impaled in the antrum displayed no slow wave activity, but slow waves in the corpus were normal in most animals. Time scales in corpus and antrum traces are the same and denoted by the black bar (1 minute). (*C*) Confocal images of Kit-like immunoreactivity in the distal (top panels) and proximal antrum (bottom panels) of nondiabetic (left panels) and diabetic (right panels) NOD mice. Note reduction in ICCs in diabetic animals. Scale bar applies to all panels. (*D*) Transmission electron micrographs of the circular muscle layers (top panels) and the myenteric regions (bottom panels) of the antrums of nondiabetic (left panels) and diabetic (right panels) NOD mice. ICCs were identified by ultrastructural features (electron-dense nucleus with heterochromatin distributed toward the periphery of the nuclear envelope, electron-dense cytoplasm, numerous mitochondria, membrane caveolae, well-developed rough endoplasmic reticulum, Golgi complexes and an incomplete basal lamina). In nondiabetic muscles intramuscular ICCs (top left panel) were closely associated with nerve fibers (*). In diabetic animals, enteric nerve fibers and bundles were not usually associated with ICCs in muscle layers (top right panel; circular muscle layer is shown). In the myenteric region, ICCs remaining in diabetic muscles (bottom right panel) were frequently separated from enteric neurons by wide extracellular spaces (ecm; G, enteroglial cell). Scale bars in control images apply to corresponding images from diabetic tissues. (Reproduced from Ordog et al., Ref. 11 with permission.)

A special category of gastric dysrhythmias may be represented by conditions that can occur in diabetes mellitus, chronic intestinal pseudo-obstruction, and aging. In these, and other, chronic conditions, structural abnormalities in ICC networks may contribute to the development of electrical dysrhythmias, much the same way that myocardial infarction affecting the conductive apparatus can lead to cardiac arrhythmias. For example, work has suggested a new hypothesis for some of the gastric emptying problems of diabetic patients. Focal disruptions of ICC networks were observed in a murine model of diabetic gastroparesis[11] (Fig. 2.8). Loss of ICCs occurred primarily in the antrum, and areas with lesions in ICC networks displayed regional loss of slow waves (Fig. 2.8). The lesion in ICC networks was not complete, and areas with normal-appearing ICCs generated slow waves at the normal frequency. It is likely that clinical evaluations that do not include region-by-region analysis of the electrical activity of the stomach might miss defects in slow waves in such patients. However, because propagation of slow waves requires regeneration of events from ICC to ICC, part of the delayed gastric emptying in diabetes may be an inability of slow waves to propagate along the normal pathway to generate gastric peristaltic contractions. Disruption of the propagation pathway could lead to conditions ranging from weakened antral contractions to a complete breakdown in coupling between the corpus and antrum. Consequences of these changes may range from relatively asymptomatic delays in gastric emptying to frank gastroparesis.

Abnormalities in slow waves were also detected in tissues with more extensive damage to the gastric ICC networks elicited by blocking cellular signaling through the receptor tyrosine kinase Kit.[3] In these animals, bradyarrhythmias and various irregular dysrhythmias (including bizarre tachybradyarrhythmias) were frequently recorded from the fringes of areas depleted of ICCs. Thus, chronic damage to ICC networks may be an important factor in some gastric dysrhythmias. It is not yet clear how isolating regions of ICC from the main pacemaker network results in remodeling of the pacemaker mechanism to produce aberrant slow wave frequencies.

More recently, the effects of structural defects on antral pacemaking were investigated using W/W^v mice, a genetic model of delayed gastric emptying.[8] Pacemaker ICCs in these mice are significantly reduced in number, particularly in the orad corpus, where large areas of the musculature lack ICCs and display no slow wave activity. The intrinsic frequency of slow waves in the antrums of these mice is abnormally elevated, approaching the frequency of the corpus. Changes in antral frequency were also manifest in ICCs isolated from W/W^v antrums, suggesting the antral arrhythmia is due to retiming of the antral pacemaker mechanism. Elevation in antral pacemaker frequency represents a form of "antral tachygastria" where the frequency of intrinsic antral pacemaking approaches the frequency of corpus pacemakers. This results in breakdown in the normal corpus-to-antrum frequency gradient. If corpus and antrum pacemakers run at similar frequencies, entrainment of antral pacemakers will be either impaired or blocked because there is insufficient time for a slow wave originating in the corpus to propagate to the antrum and drive a slow wave in this region in the proper sequence. Antral slow waves will occur independently and out of sequence, and this abnormality tends to disrupt gastric peristalsis and delay gastric emptying. Although portions of the ICC network in the antrum and corpus may remain electrically coupled, these regions of the gastric musculature become "functionally uncoupled" due to the loss of the corpus to antrum frequency gradient and failure of entrainment. Thus, W/W^v mice represent an important model of a gastric emptying disorder that may result from abnormal corpus-to-antrum entrainment. We refer to this as *functional uncoupling*, where ICC networks are present and electrically coupled but pacemaker activity cannot propagate over the normal pathway from corpus to antrum because of breakdown in the pacemaker frequency gradient. In functional uncoupling, the dominant pacemaker in the corpus cannot entrain the antral pacemakers.

Gastric arrhythmias could also be caused by neural, hormonal, or paracrine influences. Several second-messenger systems activated by biogenic compounds can alter the frequency of the pacemaking in gastric ICCs (see section on regulation of pacemaker frequency). Abnormal frequencies could result in gastric ICCs in response to a variety of biogenic substances. Abnormal responses to these substances could arise from changes in the abundance of a particular compound (and particularly if the change in abundance is restricted to one region of the stomach), changes in the receptors expressed by ICCs, or remodeling of the basic pacemaker mechanism that results in changes in the intrinsic responsiveness of pacemaker cells. Functional uncoupling of corpus and antral pacemakers could result from either enhancement in antral frequency or reduction in corpus frequency. It is interesting to note that muscarinic stimulation results in a smaller enhancement in the frequency of pacemaker activity in the corpus than in the antrum.[23] Thus, even equal stimulation of the corpus and antrum by enteric excitatory motor neurons tends to reduce the corpus-to-antrum frequency gradient. Central programming of vagal inputs to enteric excitatory neurons must regulate the outflow to corpus and antrum, and centrally induced gastric arrhythmias (as might occur in motion sickness) may result in changing the balance of neural inputs to the rhythmic regions of the stomach. It is also possible that regional production of a paracrine substance, such as prostaglandins, might result in localized changes in the intrinsic frequency of pacemaker activity. If, for example, PGE_2 was abnormally produced at a specific site in the antrum, the intrinsic frequency of pacemaker activity would be enhanced. The affected region could emerge as an ectopic, antral pacemaker and interfere with corpus-to-antrum entrainment. Localized imbalances in paracrine substances could result from acute or chronic inflammatory responses.

Cautions for the Use of Electrogastrography to Evaluate Gastric Arrhythmias

The basic concepts of gastric electrophysiology described in this chapter highlight some potential problems for the application of electrogastrography (EGG) in the clinical evaluation of gastric arrhythmias. The problem of recording gastric electrical activity from the sea of bioelectrical signals generated within the central torso of a human body is an obvious problem that other contributions to this text have considered. Gastric slow waves are relatively small-amplitude events that result from slow membrane ionic currents relative to currents flowing during nerve, cardiac, and skeletal muscle action potentials. Thus, the signals recorded with extracellular electrodes that correspond to gastric slow waves will tend to be small (200 to 500 µV) and may be masked by other, larger bioelectrical signals. EGG filters remove ultraslow rhythms, and artifacts need to be identified and excluded from analyses (see Chapter 4). The amplitude of the gastric slow wave signals is attenuated by the distance between recording electrodes on the surface of the skin and the gastric tissue producing the signal. Changes in this dimension occur naturally during respiration and gastric peristaltic contractions (i.e., the stomach indents due to contractions of the circular muscle layer during these events and pulls the active tissue away from the recording electrode). Motion artifacts due to movement of the subject may also affect the EGG recording. Electrical filtering and mathematical transformations, such as fast-Fourier transform, can solve some of these problems, as discussed in other chapters, but the "fidelity of signal" issue is always present in volume recordings of gastric electrical events.

The issue of how to evaluate coupling between the corpus and antrum is also a significant problem for single-point recordings of gastric electrical activity. The real issue in gastric electrophysiology is whether the corpus paces the distal stomach properly, because this is the basis of gastric peristalsis. For example, if the intrinsic antral frequency is abnormally elevated to levels near the intrinsic frequency of the corpus pacemaker, then there will be insufficient time for the corpus event to propagate to the antrum and entrain distal pacemakers. This leads to functional uncoupling between the pacemakers in the corpus and antrum and disrupts gastric peristalsis. This defect may be impossible to assess by recording from a single electrode, yet it could have profound effects on gastric emptying. Uncoupling between the antrum and corpus might be detectable using multichannel EGG, particularly if the antral and corpus pacemakers operate at somewhat different frequencies, but computer simulations have shown that uncoupling without frequency dissociation results in highly unpredictable patterns depending on positioning of the electrodes. The most consistent result from such recordings might be a decrease in the dominant power of the Fourier spectra.[27]

The physics and physiology of gastric pacemaker activity predict quite deleterious consequences to normal gastric peristalsis and gastric emptying if the proximal-to-distal frequency gradient, intrinsic to gastric ICC, is disrupted. As we described, this need not be an extreme change in antral or corpus frequency. Problems would be predicted if there was simple frequency matching of the intrinsic pacemakers in the corpus and antrum. This could occur if the frequency of corpus pacemakers drops to near the antral frequency or the antral frequency approaches the corpus frequency. In either case, there would be insufficient time for the corpus activity to propagate to the antrum and entrain the intrinsic pacemaker activity in this region. Functional uncoupling of the electrical activity in the corpus and antrum results in these circumstances. This specific type of uncoupling has not been described in humans. It is possible that this type of uncoupling could be missed by standard EGG procedures, although studies in humans have not been performed. Further evaluation of these possibilities in patients with gastric neuromuscular disorders is needed. Other methods (including multipoint recording) for diagnosing functional uncoupling may be useful. On the other hand, many circumstances have been defined where EGG records reveal gastric dysrhythmias such as bradygastrias and tachygastrias, as described in subsequent chapters.

Conclusions

Understanding the role of ICCs in the electrical rhythmicity of gastric muscles has greatly enhanced the ability to investigate how slow wave frequency and propagation are regulated. This will undoubtedly lead to knowledge about the mechanisms of gastric dysrhythmias at the subcellular level. We can already predict the effects of agonists and transmitters linked to certain second messengers. Points of obscurity, however, are the conditions in which biogenic agents with chronotropic effects are released, the local sources of these compounds, and the specific targeting of these agents to pacemaker cells. For example, cholinergic stimulation may have chronotropic effects on pacemaker ICCs, but do nerves in the vicinity of these cells release sufficient acetylcholine to affect frequency? PGE_2 is a potent chronotropic agent, but are there sources of prostaglandin synthesis in the vicinity of pacemaker cells? Finally, the highly plastic nature of ICCs must also be appreciated. Studies have shown that ICCs can redifferentiate and the functional phenotype can disappear and reappear depending on local tissue conditions. It is quite possible that ICCs of patients with gastric arrhythmias have altered expression of receptors, second-messenger systems, and/or molecular pacemaker components. Such changes might predispose these patients to develop gastric arrhythmias in response to normal physiological signals. It is vital to evaluate the physiology of ICCs in models of gastric arrhythmias to answer these questions.

Acknowledgments

This review and our work on gastric electrophysiology have been supported by grant (RO1-DK40569 and DK58185) from the National Institute of Kidney and Diabetes and Digestive Diseases.

References

1. Camilleri M, Malagelada J-R, Brown ML, et al: Relation between antral motility and gastric emptying of solids and liquids in humans. *Am J Physiol* 1985;249:G580–G585.
2. Dickens EJ, Hirst GDS, Tomita T: Identification of rhythmically active cells in guinea-pig stomach. *J Physiol (Lond)* 1999;514:515–531.
3. Ördög T, Ward SM, Sanders KM: Interstitial cells of Cajal generate electrical slow waves in the murine stomach. *J Physiol (Lond)* 1999;518: 257–269.
4. Szurszewski JH: Electrical basis for gastrointestinal motility. In: Johnson LR, ed. *Physiology of the Gastrointestinal Tract,* 2nd ed. New York: Raven; 1987:383–422.
5. Ozaki H, Blondfield DP, Stevens RJ, et al: Simultaneous measurement of membrane potential, cytosolic calcium and muscle tension in smooth muscle tissue. *Am J Physiol* 1991;260:C917–C925.
6. Vogalis F., Publicover NG, Hume JR, et al: Relationship between calcium current and cytosolic calcium concentration in canine gastric smooth muscle cells. *Am J Physiol* 1991;260:C1012–C1018.
7. Hightower NG, Code CF: The quantitative analysis of antral gastric motility records in normal human beings, with a study of the effects of neostigmine. Proc Mayo Clin 1950;26:697–704.
8. Ördög T, Baldo M, Danko R, et al: Plasticity of electrical pacemaking by interstitial cells of Cajal underlies gastric dysrhythmia in W/W^v mutant mice. Gastroenterology 2002;123:2028–2040.
9. El-Sharkawy TY, Morgan KG, Szurszewski JH: Intracellular electrical activity of canine and human gastric smooth muscle. *J Physiol (Lond)* 1978;279: 291–307.
10. Bauer AJ, Publicover NG, Sanders KM: Origin and spread of slow waves in canine gastric antral circular muscle. *Am J Physiol* 1985;249:G800–G806.
11. Ördög T, Takayama I, Cheung WKT, et al: Remodeling of networks of interstitial cells of Cajal in a murine model of diabetic gastroparesis. Diabetes 2000;49:1731–1739.
12. Horiguchi K, Semple GSA, Sanders KM, et al: Distribution of pacemaker function through the tunica muscularis of the canine gastric antrum. *J Physiol (Lond)* 2001;537:237–250.
13. Kim TW, Beckett EAH, Hanna R, et al: Regulation of pacemaker frequency in the murine gastric antrum. *J Physiol (Lond)* 2002A;538: 145–157.
14. Koh SD, Jun JY, Kim TW, et al: A Ca^{2+}-inhibited non-selective cation conductance contributes to pacemaker currents in cultured interstitial cells of Cajal. *J Physiol (Lond)* 2002;540:803–814.
15. Ward SM, Ördög T, Koh SD, et al: Pacemaking in interstitial cells of Cajal depends upon calcium handling by endoplasmic reticulum and mitochondria. *J Physiol (Lond)* 2000;525:355–361.

16. Sanders KM, Ördög T, Koh SD, et al: A novel pacemaker mechanism drives gastrointestinal rhythmicity. News Physiol Sci 2000;15:291–298.
17. Suzuki H, Takano H, Yamamoto Y, et al: Properties of gastric smooth muscles obtained from mice which lack inositol trisphosphate receptor. *J Physiol (Lond)* 2000;525:105–111.
18. Publicover NG, Sanders KM: A technique to locate the pacemaker in smooth muscles. *J Appl Physiol* 1984;57:1586–1590.
19. Kim YC, Koh SD, Sanders KM: Voltage-dependent inward currents of interstitial cells of Cajal from murine colon and small intestine. *J Physiol (Lond)* 2002c;541:C797–C810.
20. Nose K, Suzuki H, Kannan H: Voltage dependency of the frequency of slow waves in antrum smooth muscle of the guinea-pig stomach. *Jpn J Physiol* 2000;50:625–633.
21. Ozaki H, Blondfield DP, Hori M, et al: Cyclic AMP-mediated regulation of excitation-contraction coupling in canine gastric smooth muscle. *J Physiol (Lond)* 1992;447;351–372.
22. Tsugeno M, Huang SM, Pang YW, et al: Effects of phosphodiesterase inhibitors on spontaneous electrical activity (slow waves) in the guinea-pig gastric muscle. *J Physiol (Lond)* 1995;485:493–502.
23. Kim TW, Koh SD, Ördög T, et al: Muscarinic regulation of pacemaker frequency in gastric interstitial cells of Cajal. *J Physiol (Lond)* 2002B;in press.
24. Kim CH, Azpiroz F, Malagelada JR: Characteristics of spontaneous and drug-induced gastric dysrhythmias in a chronic canine model. Gastroenterology 1986;90:421–427.
25. Sanders KM: Role of prostaglandins in regulating gastric motility. *Am J Physiol* 1984;247:G117–G126.
26. Owyang C, Hasler WL: Physiology and pathophysiology of the interstitial cells of Cajal: from bench to bedside. VI. Pathogenesis and therapeutic approaches to human gastric dysrhythmias. *Am J Physiol* 2002; 283:8–15.
27. Liang J, Chen JDZ: What can be measured from surface electrogastrography. Dig Dis Sci 1997;42:1331–1343.

3

Physiological Basis of Electrogastrography

*I*n this chapter, the anatomical, functional, and in vivo myoelectrical characteristics of the normal stomach are reviewed. The anatomical regions of the stomach are shown in Figure 3.1. Major areas are the fundus, the body (corpus), antrum, and pyloroduodenal area. Extrinsic innervation of the stomach is provided by the vagus nerve and splanchnic nerves. The pacemaker region is shown on the greater curvature of the stomach between the fundus and the corpus. From the pacemaker region, spontaneous electrical depolarization and repolarization occurs and generates the myoelectrical waves that are termed the *gastric pacesetter potentials*, or *slow waves*.[1,2]

Gastric Pacesetter Potentials and Action Potentials

The prominent muscle layers of the stomach are the circular and the longitudinal muscle layers (see Fig. 3.1, middle). The oblique muscle layer is included in the muscularis. Between these smooth muscle layers lie the neurons of the myenteric plexus, the gastric components of

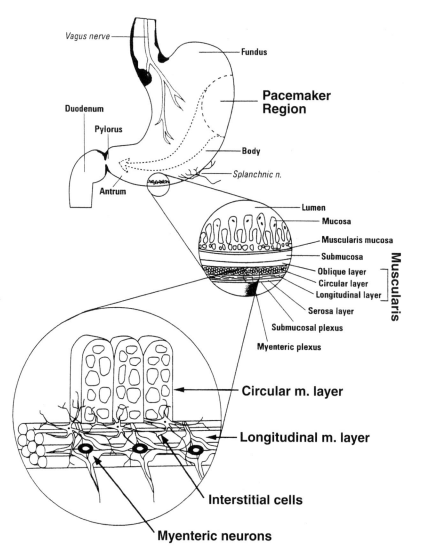

Figure 3.1. Anatomical regions of the stomach. The upper figure shows the fundus, body, and antrum of the stomach. The pacemaker region is the origin of gastric pacesetter potential activity. The cutout of the gastric wall shown in the middle portion of the figure depicts the lumen of the stomach, the mucosa, and the muscularis of the stomach wall. The main muscle layers of the stomach are the longitudinal and circular muscle layers, with some contribution by the oblique muscle layer. In the lower portion of the figure, the relationships among the circular muscle layer, the interstitial cells of Cajal, and the myenteric neurons of Auerbach's plexus are shown. The interstitial cells of Cajal synapse with the circular muscle layer as well as the myenteric neurons. The interstitial cells of Cajal are the origin of the electrical rhythmicity that is recorded as the gastric pacesetter potentials. The gastric pacesetter potentials coordinate the frequency and the propagation of the circular smooth muscle contractions.

the enteric nervous system. Afferent neurons, interneurons, and post-ganglionic parasympathetic neurons all have synaptic interactions in the myenteric plexus. Intrinsic neurons and extrinsic excitatory and inhibitory neurons from the vagus nerve and splanchnic nerves, intra-luminal contents, and hormones modulate contraction and relaxation of the smooth muscle in the different regions of the stomach.[3]

Important anatomical and functional relationships exist among the circular smooth muscle layer, the myenteric neurons, and the in-terstitial cells of Cajal (ICCs) (see Fig. 3.1, bottom). The ICCs are the pacemaker cells, the cells that spontaneously depolarize and repolar-ize and set the myoelectrical rhythmicity of the stomach and other areas of the gastrointestinal tract.[4,5] The interstitial cells are electri-cally coupled with the circular muscle cells. Low-amplitude rhythmic circular contractions occur at the pacemaker rhythm.[6] Rhythmicity and contractility of the circular muscle layer are modulated by ongoing activity excitatory and inhibitory of myenteric neurons that synapse with the interstitial cells. The interstitial cells have a variety of other receptors. Electrocontractile activities of the gastric smooth muscle are modified by neuronal and hormonal inputs appropriate for fast-ing and specific postprandial conditions. Control of rhythmicity may be modulated by a variety of stimuli that affect the interstitial cells and is a focus of intense investigation. The ICCs and control of electrical rhythmicity of the stomach are reviewed in Chapter 2.

Human gastric slow wave or pacesetter potential activity gener-ated by the ICCs occurs at a rate of 3 cycles per minute (cpm).[7-10] Pacesetter potential activity is illustrated in Figure 3.2.[8-10] Electrodes sewn onto the serosa of the stomach record the depolarization and repolarization waves of the pacesetter potentials. The electrical wave-front travels around the circumference of the stomach at a fast rate of speed and migrates slowly toward the antrum at an increasing ve-locity. As a slow wave disappears in the distal antrum, another slow wave originates in the pacemaker area and begins to migrate toward the antrum approximately every 20 seconds. When there is little smooth muscle contractility (phase I or phase II of the interdigestive state, described later), these electrical events reflect depolarization and repolarization of the ICCs and some small degree of contractility of the circular muscle cells.

From an in vivo electrical viewpoint, the fasting pacesetter po-tential activity is relatively weak compared with the gastric myoelec-trical activity during the postprandial period, when luminal contents

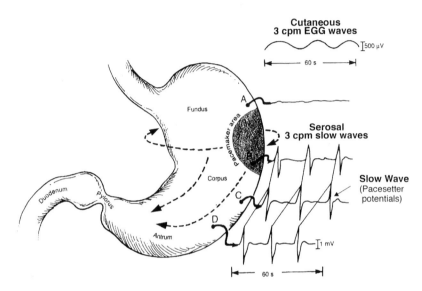

Figure 3.2. Pacesetter potentials (also termed slow waves) originate in the pacemaker region and propagate circumferentially and distally at a rate of 3 cycles per minute (cpm) (see dotted arrows). Electrical rhythmicity is not present in the fundus, as shown by the flat signal from electrode A. Sparse numbers of interstitial cells of Cajal are found in the fundus, whereas interstitial cells of Cajal densely populate the corpus and antrum. Three sequences of pacesetter potentials recorded from serosal electrodes (electrodes B, C, and D) are shown. As recorded from cutaneous electrodes, the 3-cpm waves in the electrogastrogram (EGG) reflect the sum of electrical activities occurring as the pacesetter potential sequences migrate across the corpus and antrum beneath the cutaneous electrodes. The electrical migration occurs every 20 seconds and produces 3-cpm EGG waves.

and other stimuli augment gastric neuromuscular activity.[3,11] Figure 3.3 shows a conceptualization of the human gastric pacesetter potential as an "electrical halo" migrating around the stomach very quickly and moving distally through the antrum in approximately 20 seconds resulting in the normal gastric electrical frequency of 3 cpm. As described later, it is this moving electrical wavefront that is recorded in the electrogastrogram (EGG), the gastric myoelectrical activity recorded from electrodes placed onto the surface of the epigastrium.

Additional gastric myoelectrical activity occurs when stronger circular muscle contraction occurs (e.g., when vagal efferent activity and release of acetylcholine from the postganglionic cholinergic neurons are elicited in response to ingestion of a meal). In this postprandial situation, plateau potentials and action potentials occur during circular muscle contraction (Fig. 3.4). If more action potentials or greater amplitude and duration of the plateau potentials occur, then stronger circular muscle contractions occur. Migrating circular muscle contractions may result in gentle peristaltic waves or strong lumen-obliterating contractions. Figure 3.4 shows the relationship between the pacesetter potential that is linked to the action potential or plateau potential activity and the formation of a circular muscle contraction that migrates from proximal to distal stomach. Thus, the action potential and/or the plateau potential, linked to the migrating pacesetter potential, forms the myoelectrical basis for the gastric peristaltic contractions that ultimately mix and triturate intraluminal contents. When conditions are appropriate, peristaltic contractions empty 2- to 4-ml aliquots of chyme from the stomach into the duodenum to accomplish the neuromuscular work of gastric emptying. Because of the increased gastric myoelectrical activity, the EGG signal during the postprandial peristaltic contractions is generally higher in amplitude in healthy subjects compared with the fasting EGG (Fig. 3.4).

Figure 3.5 illustrates a stronger "electrical halo" formed in the postprandial period when the additional gastric myoelectrical activity of the plateau potentials or spike potentials is linked to the migrating gastric pacesetter potential. Compared with the fasted condition (see Fig. 3.3), greater myoelectrical activity occurs at the normal 3-cpm frequency during regular peristaltic contractions (Fig. 3.5). The additional intensity of gastric myoelectrical activity is present because action potentials or plateau potentials are now linked to the ongoing gastric pacesetter potential activity. Furthermore, the electrocontractile complex

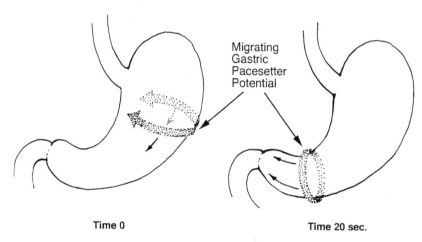

Time 0   **Time 20 sec.**

Figure 3.3. Propagation of the gastric pacesetter potential is illustrated as a faint electrical "halo." The depolarization-repolarization electrical wavefront migrates from the pacemaker region of the corpus (time 0) through the corpus to the distal antrum (time 20 seconds). These pacesetter potentials occur at approximately 3 cpm.

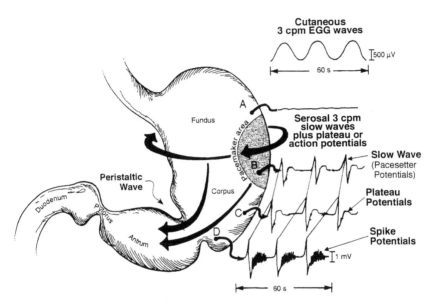

Figure 3.4. Gastric pacesetter potentials (slow waves), spike potentials and plateau potentials recorded from serosal electrodes (B, C, and D are shown). Plateau and action (spike) potentials occur during circular muscle contraction (see electrode D). When the plateau and spike potential activity are linked to the migrating pacesetter potential, a moving circular muscle contraction is formed (i.e., a gastric peristaltic wave). Arrows indicate circumferential and distal migration of the electrical and contractile activity forming a peristaltic wave.

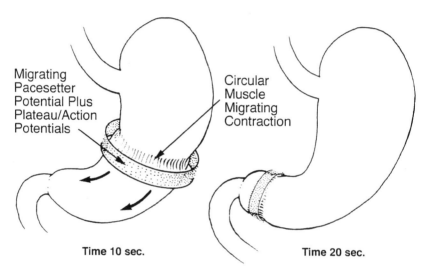

Migrating
Pacesetter
Potential Plus
Plateau/Action
Potentials

Circular
Muscle
Migrating
Contraction

Time 10 sec.

Time 20 sec.

Figure 3.5. The migration of the pacesetter potential plus plateau or action potential activity is illustrated as a stronger, moving electrical "halo" compared with
the noncontractile state (compare with Fig. 3.3). The movement of the electro-
contractile complex across the stomach is shown at 10 and 20 seconds.

(the peristaltic wave) travels circumferentially as well as distally, thus forming the stronger depolarization–repolarization wavefront (i.e., stronger "halo") shown moving through the corpus to the distal antrum where the contraction dissipates. Thus, compared with fasting, the amplitude of the EGG wave is generally greater in the postprandial condition depending on the specific meal ingested. Amplitude of the EGG signal may also be affected by the distance of the electrodes from the stomach.

These basic gastric myoelectrical activities form the physiological basis for understanding fasting and postprandial EGG patterns recorded in healthy individuals. In the later sections, the fasting and postprandial EGG patterns recorded from healthy individuals are described and illustrated in detail.

Normal Electrogastrographic Patterns in Healthy Subjects

Fasting Electrogastrographic Patterns

During prolonged fasting, the stomach and small intestine proceed through several stereotyped contraction patterns. The clearest contraction pattern is termed *phase III of the interdigestive complex.*[8] Phase III is a 3- to 10-minute period of rhythmic contractions in the antrum that migrate into the duodenum and through the small intestine to the terminal ileum every 90 to 110 min. The phase III contractions occur during prolonged fasting and thus are most readily recorded during an overnight fast. Phase I is a period of contractile quiescence that occurs in the 10 to 15 minutes after cessation of the phase III contractions. Phase II of the interdigestive complex is the 75- to 90-minute period of sporadic and inconsistent contractions of the small bowel that precedes the phase III contractions. The phase II contractions increase in frequency near the initiation of phase III contractions.

The EGG correlates of the interdigestive complex in the stomach have been described.[12] The clearest 3-cpm EGG signals generally occur during phase I, when there is contractile quiescence, at least as measured by intraluminal pressure catheters. At this time, the 3-cpm EGG activity is the most stable and likely reflects the underlying activity of the ICCs. During phase II, when contractions are irregular, the 3-cpm EGG signal is more unstable. During phase III contractions, 3-cpm EGG waves may have increased amplitude (Fig. 3.6). However,

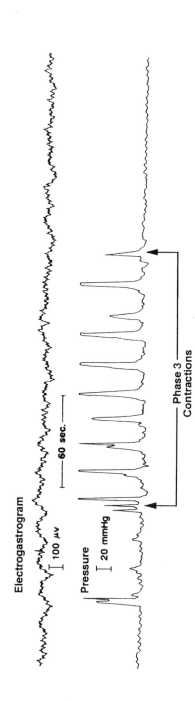

Figure 3.6. Electrogastrogram (EGG) rhythm strip and intraluminal pressure in the antrum recorded during fasting from a healthy subject. The EGG signal shows slight increase in amplitude of 3-cpm activity at the same time that phase 3 contractions are recorded during the interdigestive state.

clear increase in the amplitude of 3-cpm EGG waves occurred only 50% of the time when phase III contractions are present.[12] Thus, increased amplitude of the EGG signal during fasting does not reliably reflect the presence of phase III contractions.

In general, the EGG signal recorded when the stomach is empty is usually a low-amplitude 3-cpm rhythm or unstable signal that may vary from the 3-cpm normal range (2.5–3.7 cpm) to tachygastria (3.7–10.0 cpm) and bradygastria (1.0–2.5 cpm) ranges. For these reasons, investigators have used a variety of meals and drugs to stimulate the fasted or baseline gastric myoelectrical activity. The next section reviews postprandial EGG patterns in healthy individuals.

Postprandial Electrogastrographic Patterns

The stomach must respond appropriately to a vast variety of intraluminal stimuli. In addition, the stomach reacts to visual, olfactory, and gustatory stimuli during the cephalic phase of digestion. The stomach neuromuscular apparatus initially responds to the ingestion of solid foods and liquids with relaxation of the gastric muscular wall of the fundus.[3] The fundus relaxes to receive the volume of food ingested. This important phenomenon is called *receptive relaxation* and is illustrated in Figure 3.7. Receptive relaxation is a vagally mediated event mediated by nitric oxide. The nitric oxide–triggered relaxation of the fundus and proximal corpus allows the stomach to receive the ingested volume of food without increasing intragastric pressures or inducing excessive stretch (tension) on the gastric muscle walls.[3,13] Stretch or tension of the gastric walls stimulates vagal afferent nerve activity, which may be perceived by an individual as fullness or discomfort, postprandial perceptions or symptoms that are discussed in later chapters.

Solid food is emptied from the fundus into the corpus antrum and mixed with acid and pepsin (see Fig. 3.7). The distal corpus and antrum do not relax or stretch to the same degree as the fundus. The corpus antrum is the main mixing chamber for the trituration of ingested solid foods. Recurrent gastric peristaltic contractions gently break down the solid foods (trituration) and form chyme, a nutrient suspension with particles 1 to 2 mm in diameter.[3,13] Chyme is pumped into the duodenum through the pylorus in 2- to 4-ml aliquots by the recurrent gastric peristaltic waves (antral systole).[14] The pylorus and duodenal contractions provide resistance to flow and modulate the

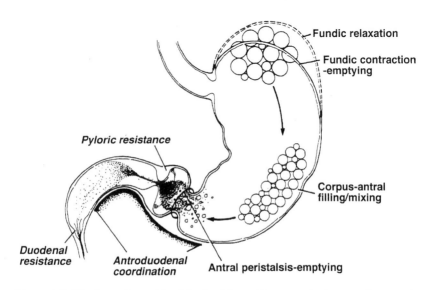

Figure 3.7. The ingestion of food by healthy subjects results in complex gastric neuromuscular responses: Those responses include receptive relaxation of proximal stomach (fundus), emptying and distribution of the ingested solid food into the corpus antrum, corpus antrum mixing and trituration, emptying of chyme by antral peristalsis that is modulated by antroduodenal coordination, and pyloric and duodenal resistances.

rate of gastric emptying.[3] The neuromuscular work of the stomach is applied to the ingested food by the electrocontractile activities produced by pacesetter potentials linked with the action and plateau potentials. These electrocontractile relationships are described here.

Liquids are emptied by recurrent gastric peristaltic waves in a pulsatile manner as shown by nuclear medicine studies and ultrasonographic studies.[15,16] In some circumstances, liquids are also emptied through the pylorus in the absence of peristaltic waves through the establishment of a pressure gradient between the stomach and the duodenum.[12] Orange juice or water empty exponentially compared with solid foods, which have a variable lag phase followed by a linear emptying phase. However, liquids with high caloric content or highly viscous liquids empty slowly from the stomach in patterns that resemble the emptying of solid food.[3]

The relationships between the emptying of barium from the stomach and gastric electrical events recorded from a healthy subject are shown in Figure 3.8. The fluoroscopic images of the stomach show that barium suspension is emptied from the corpus antrum into the duodenum by a peristaltic contraction. Sequential radiographs of the stomach during a gastric peristaltic wave are shown in frames 1, 2, 3 and 4. The asterisk indicates EGG recording electrodes positioned on the epigastrium. The small, black arrows indicate a circular muscle contraction that is migrating through the antrum (frames 1 and 2) and begins to empty barium into the duodenal bulb (frames 3 and 4). EGG wave A with frames 1, 2, 3, and 4 was recorded during the progression of the gastric peristaltic wave shown by the radiographs in frames 1 to 4.[17] During the gastric peristaltic wave, the EGG wave peaked (see 2 on EGG wave A) and then the amplitude decreased (see 4 on EGG wave A). EGG wave B was recorded during the next gastric peristaltic wave, which is shown in the radiographs in frames 5, 6, and 7. This peristaltic wave also emptied barium into the duodenal bulb as shown in frame 7. Thus, each gastric peristaltic wave emptied a small aliquot of the barium from the antrum into the duodenal bulb.[17] One EGG wave reflected the myoelectrical activity of a peristaltic wave that migrated from proximal to distal stomach. This sequence repeated itself until the noncaloric barium meal was emptied from the stomach.

The important point is that each EGG wave is a summary of the electrical events that occur during a barium-induced peristaltic wave. The peristaltic wave is the "electrical halo" described earlier that is

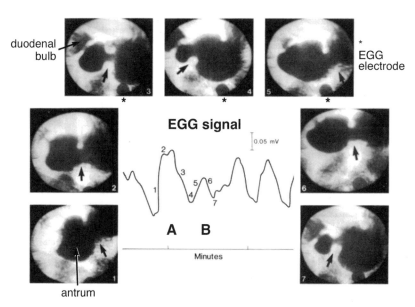

Figure 3.8. Simultaneous electrogastrogram (EGG) recording and fluoroscopic imaging of the barium-filled stomach in a healthy subject. Each EGG wave (*A* and *B*) correlated with a gastric peristaltic contraction (see radiographic frames 1–4 and 5–7). The small black arrow indicates the migrating peristaltic contraction. Each of the peristaltic waves emptied an aliquot of barium into the duodenum (see frames 3 and 7). These electrocontractile waves are examples of "antral systole." *One EGG electrode. (See text for details.)

formed as the pacesetter potential linked to plateau or spike potential moves from the corpus to the pylorus beneath the recording electrodes. Thus, the EGG signal as recorded by surface electrodes after a barium meal, a provocative water load test, or a caloric meal reflects the gastric pacesetter potential activity (ICC activity) *and* the myoelectrical activity associated with circular muscle contraction (action and plateau potentials). These are the electrical events that produce *gastric peristalsis*, the peristaltic contractions that produce emptying of the barium meal.

Electrodes placed on the epigastrium along the axis of the antrum record the sum of rhythmic electrical events produced by the gastric pacesetter potentials and action/plateau potentials that migrate across the stomach from the pacemaker region to the antrum (Fig. 3.9). With proper filtering and standard test protocols (and proper recording and analysis methods, as discussed in Chapters 4 and 5), reliable EGGs and EGG responses to various stimuli can be recorded for physiological and clinical studies.[7]

The water load test, for example, is a provocative test that stimulates the neuromuscular activity of the stomach as the subject ingests a noncaloric physical volume of water. Water is ingested over a 5-minute period. The muscle tone from the fundus to the antrum initially relaxes to receive the volume of water. The stomach then develops recurrent peristaltic contractions to empty the liquid from the stomach. Ultrasonographic studies indicate that the ingestion of 500 ml of a brothy liquid results in a dramatic increase in the volume of the stomach from less than 50 ml at fasting baseline to 353 ml at 10 minutes after ingestion. The liquid meal distended the antrum, corpus, and fundus.[18] Figure 3.10 illustrates the physical distention of the antrum, corpus, and fundus and gastric myoelectrical activity after the water load test. In this example, the healthy subject has a fasting stomach volume of 50 ml and 3-cpm myoelectrical activity is recorded from serosal electrodes and in the EGG signal. The healthy subject ingests 500 ml of water, the stomach distends normally (i.e., normal muscle relaxation or stretch), and normal 3-cpm EGG activity is evoked as shown by the serosal and EGG recordings. The amplitude of the electrical waves increases after the water load. The water load test and EGG activity in a healthy subject are contrasted with results from patients with unexplained nausea in later chapters.

The standard water load test with EGG recording is outlined in Figure 3.11. After an overnight fast, a 200-Kcal meal of toast and

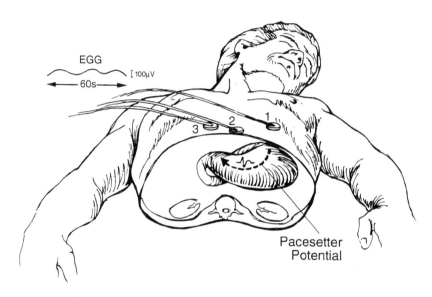

Figure 3.9. Illustration of gastric pacesetter potential activity migrating distally across the stomach surface and electrodes positioned on the epigastrium to record gastric myoelectrical activity, the electrogastrogram (EGG). The EGG records the frequency and amplitude of the electrical events beneath the electrodes.

Healthy Subject

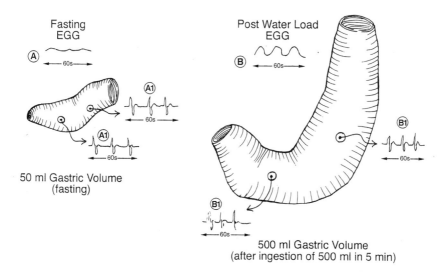

Fasting
EGG

Post Water Load
EGG

50 ml Gastric Volume
(fasting)

500 ml Gastric Volume
(after ingestion of 500 ml in 5 min)

Figure 3.10. Illustration of the stomach volume and myoelectrical activity during fasting (A) and after ingestion of water until full (B). The 3-cpm gastric myoelectrical activity is recorded from the corpus and antrum by serosal and electrogastrogram (EGG) electrodes. The EGG shows 3-cpm signal during fasting and increased amplitude of the 3-cpm signal after the water load. Note the 10-fold increase in gastric capacity after the water load, a response requiring relaxation of the musculature before commencement of muscular contraction activity for emptying. In this healthy subject, the EGG rhythm remains in a 3-cpm pattern after the water load.

EGG with Water Load Test

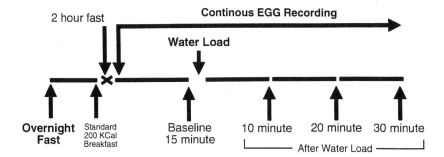

Figure 3.11. Electrogastrogram (EGG) recording and the water load test. The water load test involves the ingestion of water over a 5-minute period until the subject "feels full." Visual analog scales may be used to assess visceral perceptions or symptoms during these periods.

apple juice is given. The subject then fasts an additional 2 hours after the premeal to ensure a stable and controlled 15-minute baseline EGG recording. After a 15-minute baseline EGG is recorded, the subject is asked to drink until "full" over a 5-minute period from a 1-L container of water (23°C). The EGG is recorded for 30 minutes after ingestion of the water. Then the baseline and three consecutive 10-minute periods of EGG recordings after the water load are analyzed. The volume of water ingested in 5 minutes, indicating gastric volume or capacity, is recorded.

In response to the water load, there is a predictable pattern of EGG responses in healthy individuals.[19] The baseline EGG rhythm usually shifts to a 1- to 2-cpm bradygastria rhythm during the first 10 minutes after the ingestion of water. The "frequency dip" is also seen initially after the ingestion of cold water (not body temperature water) and after yogurt meals.[20] By 20 and 30 minutes after ingestion of the water, the 3-cpm EGG rhythm begins to dominate the EGG signal. The 3-cpm EGG waves are generally greater in amplitude 20 minutes after ingestion compared with baseline. In many subjects, the 3-cpm rhythm continues to increase in amplitude by 30 minutes after ingestion of the water compared with baseline. In other subjects, there is some decrease in 3-cpm activity by the 30-minute point. Symptoms such as nausea, bloating, and stomach fullness are recorded on a visual analog scale before and after the water load test.

The water load test evokes pure stomach neuromuscular activity without the influence of olfactory, visual, or gustatory cues of a caloric meal. The response of the stomach is the neuromuscular activity (relaxation or stretch followed by contractions) induced by the volume of the ingested water. There are no confounding effects on the stomach induced by increases in cholecystokinin, secretin, or insulin that occur after the ingestion of a meal containing fat, carbohydrate, or protein, respectively.[3]

An EGG recorded from a healthy person during the water load test is shown in Figure 3.12. The insets show the EGG rhythm strip at baseline (A) and approximately 20 minutes after ingestion of the water load (B). The baseline EGG shows some 3-cpm activity, and after the ingestion of water, there are 3-cpm EGG waves with increased amplitude. Figure 3.12 also shows the running spectral analysis (RSA), an analysis of the frequencies in the EGG signal. The X-axis indicates the frequencies contained in the EGG signal from 0 to 15 cpm. The Y-axis indicates time, with each line comprising 4 minutes of EGG

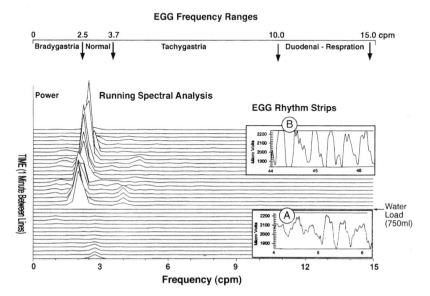

Figure 3.12. Electrogastrogram (EGG) recording and running spectral analysis (RSA) before and after the water load test in a healthy subject. The EGG rhythm strips are from before (A) and after (B) the water load. Water load test time is indicated by the arrow and two flat lines in the running spectral analysis (RSA). The X-axis indicates frequency from 0 to 15 cpm, the Y-axis indicates time, and the Z-axis or three-dimensional looking peaks indicate the strength or the power of the frequencies in the raw EGG signal. At the top of the figure, the frequencies of the four relevant ranges are shown: bradygastria (0–2.5 cpm), normal (2.5–3.7 cpm), tachygastria (3.7–10.0 cpm), and duodenal respiration (10–15 cpm). This subject shows a good 3-cpm response to the water load (EGG rhythm strip B) and concordant strong peaks at 3 cpm in the RSA (B1) after the water load.

data with a 75% overlap. Thus, each new line represents 1 new minute of EGG data added to the previous 3 minutes of EGG data. Finally, the third dimension, or Z-axis, indicates the power of the different frequencies (from 0 to 15 cpm) that are contained in the EGG signal. Details of the RSA are reviewed in Chapter 5.

In this RSA, several small peaks are seen at 3 cpm during the baseline before the water load A1 in (Fig. 3.12). The water load period is indicated at the right margin of the figure (arrow). This patient ingested 750 ml during the water load test (healthy individuals ingest approximately 600 ml). After ingestion of the water, there are clear peaks in the RSA initially at 2 cpm and then the peaks evolve toward 3 cpm by the end of the recording (B2). This is a normal EGG response and normal water load test by volume ingested.

At the top of the figure, the ranges of normal EGG activity are listed. The normal gastric pacesetter activity ranges from 2.5 to 3.7 cpm and reflects the mean normal frequency ± 2 SD.[21–24] Based on recordings from serosal recordings bradygastrias range from 0 to 2.5 cpm and tachygastrias from 3.7 to 10.0 cpm. The duodenal pacesetter frequency potential is approximately 12 to 13 cpm. In some individuals, respiration can be very slow and enter into the duodenal and even tachygastria range. Thus, the 10- to 15-cpm range is termed the *duodenal-respiration range.* Throughout this chapter, the raw EGG signal and the RSA of the EGG signal are presented in this format.

Additional examples of EGG responses recorded from healthy subjects in response to the water load are shown in Figures 3.13 to 3.15. EGG rhythm strips, the RSA, and the percentage distribution of EGG power from 1 to 15 cpm are used for clinical interpretation of gastric myoelectrical activity. There is some variability in the normal EGG response to the water load, as shown in the examples. An EGG pattern with an initial frequency dip and then 3-cpm peaks after the water load is shown in Figure 3.13. The baseline EGG signal shows some 3-cpm waves (A). After ingestion of water, there is higher-amplitude 3-cpm EGG activity in the rhythm strip. The smaller notched waves seen in the EGG waves are from respiration that is occurring at approximately 13 cpm. The 3-cpm EGG waves may also carry respiratory waves indicative of contractions of the diaphragm. The RSA shows peaks at 3 cpm at baseline. The water load period is indicated. This subject ingested 550 mL of water. After the ingestion of water, there are increased peaks at 2 cpm, the "frequency dip" that is seen after the ingestion of most liquid meals. After approximately

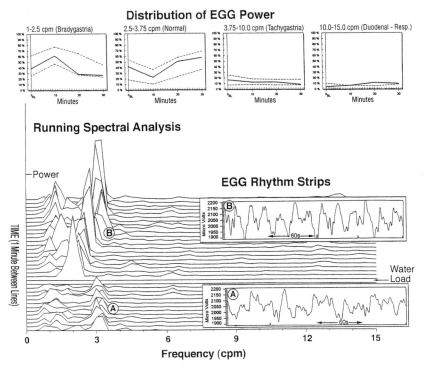

Figure 3.13. The electrogastrogram (EGG) rhythm strips, running spectral analysis (RSA), and percentage distribution of EGG power with a temporary "frequency dip" after the water load. The EGG rhythm strip recorded from a healthy subject shows clearer 3-cpm EGG waves after the water load (B) compared with baseline (A). The RSA shows 3-cpm peaks at baseline (A), a frequency dip to 2-cpm peaks initially after the water load, and then later in the analysis, 3-cpm peaks of greater amplitude (B). The percentage distribution of EGG power graphs show the normal response to the water load test. (See text for details.)

10 minutes, increasing peaks at 3 cpm are seen. Thus, this is a normal EGG response to a water load.

Also shown in Figure 3.13 are graphs of the percentage distribution of EGG power in the four frequency ranges of relevance described earlier. The dashed lines indicate the normal range of percentages at baseline and at 10, 20, and 30 minutes after the water load test. Baseline period is indicated as BL. A decrease in the percentage of EGG power in the normal 3-cpm range is seen at 10 minutes after the ingestion of water. The percentage of EGG power in the normal range then steadily increases 20 and 30 minutes after the water load. On the other hand, after ingestion of water, the percentage of EGG power in the bradygastria range increases at 10 minutes. (This increase in bradygastria power reflects the 'frequency dip' that occurs initially after the ingestion of cool water.) In the 20 and 30 minutes after the ingestion of water, the percentage of power in the bradygastria range decreases. Also shown is the percentage of power in the tachygastria range, which remains less than 20%, and there is a very low percentage of power in the duodenal respiration range (less than 10%). Overall, the percent distributions of EGG power at baseline and in response to the water load of 550 ml of water are within the normal range, as shown by the black line indicating the subject's results. Thus, inspection of the raw EGG signal, the RSA pattern, and the percentage distribution of EGG power allows for interpretation and diagnosis of the EGG recording.

A strong 3-cpm response to the water load is shown in Figure 3.14. The baseline EGG recordings shows unstable EGG waves; after ingestion of water (B), the EGG shows regular 3-cpm waves. The RSA in this subject shows some peaks at 3 cpm during baseline and increased 3-cpm peaks after the water load. The subject ingested 620 ml of water. After the ingestion of water, there is a period of flat lines with small peaks at 2 cpm. This is another example of the frequency dip response that occurs initially after the ingestion of water. Subsequently, the peaks in the RSA in the normal 3-cpm range progressively increase in power (B).

The percent *distribution of EGG power* in the four frequency ranges is also shown after the ingestion of water. At baseline, the percent distribution of power in each of the four frequency ranges is within the normal range. The pattern of EGG activity after the water load can be observed in these panels: initially the normal 3-cpm activity decreases at 10 minutes, but it increases in the normal range at

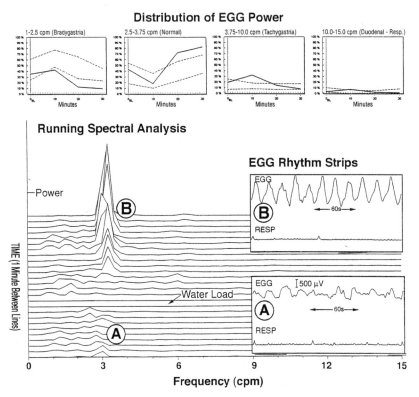

Figure 3.14. Electrogastrogram (EGG) rhythm strips, running spectral analysis (RSA), and percentage distribution of EGG power in a normal subject. The EGG rhythm strip shows some 3-cpm activity at baseline (A). RESP indicates respiratory signal. After ingestion of water, very clear regular 3-cpm waves are seen in the rhythm strip (B). The RSA shows low-power peaks at 3 cpm at baseline (A). In the first few minutes after the water load, a few small peaks are seen at 2 and 6 cpm, but then 3-cpm peaks with increasing power are seen in the RSA (B). The percentage distribution of EGG power graphs shows a normal pattern of response in the 3-cpm range with a slight and temporary increase in tachygastria 10 minutes after the ingestion of water. Overall, this is a normal EGG and water load test. (See text for details.)

20 and 30 minutes after the ingestion of water. Bradygastria power is low during each period in this subject, but there is a transient increase in tachygastria at the 10-minute point when the stomach is full of water. However, the overall percent distribution of EGG power in the 3-cpm percentages is normal at 10, 20, and 30 minutes. after the water load. Overall, this is a normal EGG and water load recording.

Figure 3.15 shows an example of an EGG with weak baseline 3-cpm activity and a good 3-cpm response to the water load. The EGG shows low-amplitude signals at baseline (A), and thus 3-cpm activity is difficult to define by visual inspection. After the ingestion of water, however, there are clear 3-cpm EGG waves (B). The RSA shows low power peaks at 1 to 2 cpm and at 3 cpm during baseline (A). At the point where the water load is indicated, this subject ingested 590 ml of water. After the ingestion of water, there was a slight decrease in EGG frequency to approximately 2.2 cpm for several minutes, and then increasing peaks in the normal 3-cpm range are seen (B). The percent distribution of EGG power graphs show normal baseline and strong 3-cpm responses after the ingestion of water. Furthermore, the percent distribution of EGG power in the bradygastria and tachygastria ranges are within the normal range for the EGG and water load test. Thus, overall this is a normal EGG with water load test.

This RSA in Figure 3.15 is presented because there are peaks at approximately 4.5 cpm and then approximately 6 cpm at the end of the recording. These smaller peaks represent harmonics of the primary frequencies of 2.2 and 3 cpm. Harmonics are generated by the Fast-Fourier transform when the shape of the raw signal is less sinusoidal and more pointed. Harmonics should not be confused with tachygastrias. See Chapter 4 for a further discussion of harmonics in the RSA.

Tachygastrias generally do not occur when the 3-cpm EGG activity is strong as seen in the rhythm strip (see Fig. 3.15). Thus, as a check for tachygastrias, the raw EGG signal must be inspected visually to see if a 6-cpm tachygastria is actually present. As shown in the EGG (inset B), no 6-cpm EGG activity is present. Therefore, the smaller peaks in the RSA at 4.5 and 6 cpm are harmonics of the 3-cpm primary frequency and do not represent tachygastrias.

The water load test has been well characterized in healthy individuals and forms a practical basis on which to assess gastric neuromuscular activity in patients with a variety of symptoms such as nausea and dysmotility-like dyspepsia symptoms.[19] The normal EGG response

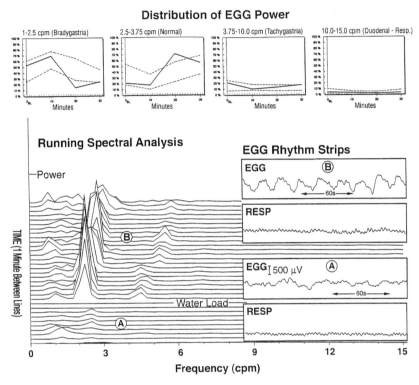

Figure 3.15. Electrogastrogram (EGG) rhythm strips, running spectral analysis (RSA), and percentage distribution of EGG power in a healthy subject. Normal 3-cpm waves are seen in the EGG rhythm strips (A and B). Respiration (Resp) signals are also shown in this example. The 3-cpm peaks at 2.5 and 3 cpm are seen in the RSA at (B) after the water load. The small peaks at 5 and 6 cpm after the water load are harmonics of the primary frequencies 2.5 and 3 cpm. Normal percentage distribution of EGG power before and after the water load test is also shown. This is a normal EGG and water load test. (See text for details.)

to a water load test in healthy subjects is contrasted with gastric dys-rhythmias recorded from patients with nausea and dyspepsia symp-toms in Chapters 6 through 8.

The EGG pattern before and after a healthy subject ingested a 220-Kcal soup meal containing various vegetables is shown in Figure 3.16. The soup meals were more filling and reduced hunger more completely than did drinking water until full. Furthermore, the soup meal induced an EGG pattern that was remarkable in that both 3- and 6–7-cpm EGG activity were seen. The 3-cpm activity predomi-nates in healthy individuals after ingestion of the soup meal. The 6-cpm activity that occurred was not a harmonic but rather was an intermittent 6-cpm tachygastria. Postprandial tachygastrias after the soup meal may represent a "physiological tachygastria" that may (1) normally slow the rate of emptying of the meal and/or (2) represent peripheral (i.e., gastric) physiological events that are perceived as in-creased fullness or satiety (not nausea) by these healthy subjects.[25]

An additional factor that can affect EGG recordings is the cephalic phase of digestion. During the cephalic phase, vagal activity stimulates gastric acid secretion and contractions before the inges-tion of foodstuffs. In a series of experiments performed by Stern et al.,[26, 27] a sham feeding protocol was designed to stimulate cephalic vagal activity. Cephalic vagal stimulation induced by sham feeding resulted in an increase in the amplitude of 3-cpm activity, as shown in Figure 3.17A. When the same food (a hot dog on a bun) was then in-gested, the expected increase in 3-cpm EGG activity occurred as the postprandial gastric neuromuscular activity commenced. Of note, patients with vagotomy did not develop increased 3-cpm EGG activity during sham feeding.

On the other hand, in healthy subjects who found the sham feed-ing procedure "disgusting," there was *no* increase in the 3-cpm EGG activity during sham feeding.[28] This failure of EGG response during "disgust" associated with sham feeding is shown in Figure 3.17B. Thus, the increase in 3-cpm EGG activity during sham feeding is normally mediated via vagal afferent activity, but the subject's negative appraisal of the food at the time of eating attenuated the gastric electrical re-sponse in the subjects who thought that the sham feeding procedure was a disgusting experience.[24] These observations may have relevance to normal eating behaviors and eating disorders.

To summarize, the EGG signal reflects gastric pacesetter activity with or without plateau or spike potential activity. The EGG signal is

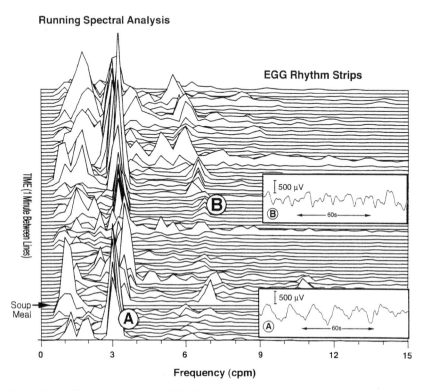

Figure 3.16. Electrogastrogram (EGG) rhythm strips and running spectral analysis (RSA) of the EGG signal before and for 2 hours after ingestion of a 220-Kcal soup meal. The EGG strip (A) shows clear 3-cpm waves before the meal at baseline. EGG strip after the soup meal (B) shows 7-cpm tachygastria. The RSA at (A) shows peaks at 3 cpm before ingestion of the soup. After ingestion of soup, 3-cpm peaks increase for almost 2 hours. Approximately 7-cpm peaks are also seen after ingestion of the soup as located at (B) on the RSA. Inspection of the raw EGG signal (B) indicated that these 7-cpm peaks reflect tachygastria signals that developed after this meal.

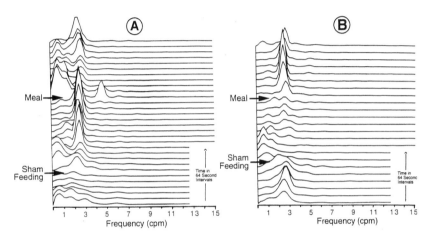

Figure 3.17. (A) Running spectral analysis (RSA) of the electrogastrogram (EGG) signal recorded from a healthy subject before and after sham feeding induced by chewing and spitting out a hot dog on a bun. Before the sham feeding, there are very few 3-cpm peaks in the RSA. During sham feeding, the 3-cpm peaks clearly increase. At the end of sham feeding, the subject ingested a meal (hot dog on a bun) and an increase in 3-cpm peaks is seen after consumption of the meal. (B) RSA of the EGG signal recorded from a different healthy individual during sham feeding. At baseline before sham feeding, 3-cpm peaks are seen, but during sham feeding, no increase in 3-cpm EGG peaks is noted. This person reported that the sham feeding process was "disgusting." When the subject ingested the meal (hot dog on a bun), however, normal 3-cpm peaks developed.

affected by a variety of cephalic-phase or meal-related stimuli. The physiological basis of the EGG signal provides the background for interpreting gastric dysrhythmias discussed in Chapters 6 through 8. In Chapters 4 and 5, EGG recording and analysis methods are reviewed.

References

1. Koch KL, Stern RM: Functional disorders of the stomach. *Semin Gastrointest Disease* 1996;4:185–195.

2. Hinder RA, Kelley KA: Human gastric pacesetter potential: sight of origin, spread, and response to gastric transection and proximal vagotomy. *Am J Surg* 1997;133:29–33.

3. Lin HC, Hasler WL: Disorders of gastric emptying. In: Yamada T, ed. *Textbook of Gastroenterology*. Philadelphia: JB Lippincott;1995:1318–1346.

4. Thunberg L: Interstitial cells of Cajal. In: Wood JD, ed. *The Handbook of Physiology, The Gastrointestinal System,* Section 6, Vol 1, Part 1. Bethesda, MD: American Physiological Society 1989:349–386.

5. Huisinga JD: Physiology and pathophysiology of the interstitial cell of Cajal: From bench to bedside, II: gastric motility: lessons from mutant mice on slow waves and innervation. *Am J Physiol* 2001;281:G1129–G1134.

6. Kim TW, Beckett EAH, Hanna R, et al: Regulation of pacemaker frequency in the murine gastric antrum. *J Physiol* (Lond) 2002;538:145–157.

7. Koch KL: The stomach: electrogastrography. In: Schuster M, Crowell M, and Koch KL, eds. *Atlas of Gastrointestinal Motility*. Ontario, Canada: BC Decker; 2002:185–201.

8. Szurzewski JH: Electrical basis for gastrointestinal motility. In: Johnson LR, ed. *Physiology of the Gastrointestinal Tract,* 2nd ed. New York: Raven; 1987:383–422.

9. Hamilton JW, Bellahsene BE, Reicherlderfer M, et al: Human electrogastrograms. Comparison of surface and mucosal recordings. Dig Dis Sci 1986;31:33–39.

10. You CH, Lee KY, Chey WY, et al: Electrogastrographic study of patients with unexplained nausea, bloating and vomiting. *Gastroenterology* 1980; 79:311–314.

11. Lacey BE, Koch KL, Crowell MD: The stomach: normal function and clinical disorders. Manometry. In: Schuster M, Crowell M, Koch KL, eds. *Atlas of Gastrointestinal Motility*. Ontario, Canada: BC Decker;2002: 135–150.

12. Meyer JE: Motility of the stomach in gastroduodenal junction. In: *Physiology of the Gastrointestinal Tract*. Ed. LR Johnson, Raven Press, New York, NY, 1987:393–410.

13. Geldof H, van der Schee EJ, Grashuis JL: Electrogastrographic charac-
    teristics of the interdigestive migrating complex in humans. Am J Phys-
    iol 1986;250:G165–G171.
14. Malbert CH, Ruckebusch Y: Relationships between pressure and flow
    across the gastroduodenal junction in dogs. Am J Physiol 1991;260:
    G653–G657.
15. Bolondi L, Bortolotti MS, Calleti T, et al: Measurement of gastric empty-
    ing by real-time ultrasonography. Gastroenterology 1985;89:752–759.
16. Urbain JL, VanCutsem E, Siegel JA, et al: Visualization and characteriza-
    tion of gastric contractions using a radionuclide technique. Am J Physiol
    1990;259:G1062–G1067.
17. Koch KL, Stewart WR, Stern RM: Effect of barium meals on gastric
    electromechanical activity in man. A fluoroscopic-electrogastrographic
    study. Dig Dis Sci 1987;32:1217–1222.
18. Gilja OH, Detmer PR, Jong JM, et al: Intragastric distribution and gas-
    tric emptying assessed by three-dimensional ultrasonography. Gastroen-
    terology 1997;113:38–49.
19. Koch KL, Hong S-P, Xu L: Reproducibility of gastric myoelectrical activ-
    ity and the water load test in patients with dysmotility-like dyspepsia
    symptoms and in control subjects. J Clin Gastroenterol 2000;31:125–129.
20. ver Hagen MA, Luijk HC, Samson M, et al: Effect of meal temperature
    on the frequency of gastric myoelectrical activity. Neurogastroenterol Motil
    1998;10:175–181.
21. Hinder RA, Kelly KA: Human gastric pacesetter potential. Site of origin,
    spread, and response to gastric transsection and proximal gastric vago-
    tomy. Am J Surg 1997;133:29–33.
22. You CH, Chey WY, Lee KY, et al: Gastric and small intestinal myoelectri-
    cal dysrhythmia associated with chronic intractable nausea and vomit-
    ing. Ann Intern Med 1981;95:449–453.
23. Hamilton JW, Bellahsene BE, Reichelderfer M, et al: Human electrogas-
    trograms. Comparison of surface and mucosal recordings. Dig Dis Sci
    1986;31:33–39.
24. Lin C, Chen JDZ, Schirmer BD, et al: Postprandial response of gastric
    slow waves: correlation of serosal recordings with the electrogastrogram.
    Dig Dis Sci 2000;45:645–651.
25. Xu L, Koch KL, Gianaros PJ, et al: The effects of soup, casserole, and wa-
    ter ingestion on gastric myoelectrical activity and perception of hunger
    and fullness. Am J Gastroenterol 2002;122:326A.
26. Stern RM, Crawford HE, Stewart W, et al: Sham feeding: cephalic-vagal
    influences on gastric myoelectrical activity. Dig Dis Sci 1989;34:521–527.
27. Stern RM, Jokerst MD, Levine ME, et al: The stomach's response to un-
    appetizing food: cephalic-vagal effects on gastric myoelectrical activity.
    Neurogastroenterol Motil 2001;13:1–4.

4

Recording the Electrogastrogram

*E*lectrogastrograms (EGGs) are recorded by placing electro-cardiogram (ECG)-type electrodes on the surface of the epi-gastrium. The EGG is one of several biological signals that can be recorded from the electrodes on the epigastrium. Some of these signals, like the ECG, are much stronger than the EGG. The EGG signal is relatively low amplitude, ranging from approximately 100 to 500 µV. Thus, the EGG signal must be properly amplified and filtered for quality recordings. To reduce baseline drift and to re-move unwanted cardiac and respiratory signals, a 0.016-Hz high-pass filter and a 0.25-Hz low-pass filter are used. These filters create a bandpass, or window, from approximately 1 cycle per minute (cpm) to 15 cpm through which the desired gastric myoelectrical signals pass during the EGG recording.

In this chapter, the equipment needed to record the EGG, the EGG recording procedure, and how to identify and reduce artifacts in EGG recordings are discussed. For additional information on the acquisition and analysis of EGG data, the reader is referred to several reviews and texts.[1-3]

Equipment

Electrodes

High-quality, fresh, disposable electrodes such as those used for electrocardiogram (ECG) recording are recommended. To minimize artifacts in the EGG recording caused by electrode movement on the skin, it is best to use electrodes that adhere very well to the skin (e.g., Cleartrace; ConMed Corp., Utica, NY; or BioTac; Graphic Controls, Inc., Buffalo, NY). Reusable silver/silver chloride electrodes are available (e.g., 1081 Biode; UFI, Morro Bay, CA). The size of the electrode surface is not important, but the electrical stability of the electrode is important. The electrodes should show little bias or offset potential because the EGG signal is relatively low amplitude and low frequency.

Recording Equipment

A high-quality recording system is needed to amplify and process the 100 to 500-μV EGG signal that ranges from 1.0 to 15.0 cpm. Some older physiological polygraphs have appropriate amplifiers and filters that can be used to record the EGG. Several medical device companies produce complete EGG recording and analysis systems that include appropriate amplifiers and filters with analog-to-digital boards that digitize the EGG signal for analysis with software (e.g., 3CPM Company, Crystal Bay, NV; Medtronic, Shoreview, MN). The 3CPM Company and Medtronic, Inc. EGG hardware and analysis software are approved by the Food and Drug Administration for clinical use for the diagnosis of gastric dysrhythmias. Ambulatory EGG equipment is also available, and data are stored on a RAM card for later analysis (UFI, Morro Bay, CA). A visual display of the raw EGG signal is very important to select artifact-free EGG signal for visual or computer analysis.

Recording Procedure

Electrode Placement

Electrodes are placed on the skin surface of the epigastrium over the general area of the corpus and antrum of the stomach. EGGs are obtained with electrodes arranged for bipolar recordings. A reference electrode is positioned on the right side of the patient's abdomen. The approximate position of the electrodes relative to the umbilicus and ribs is shown in Figure 4.1. One active electrode should be placed approximately 10 cm cephalad from the umbilicus and 6 cm to the patient's left. It is important to place this electrode below, and not on, the lowest rib to avoid respiratory signals. The second active electrode should be placed approximately 4 cm above the umbilicus (midway between the umbilicus and xiphoid) on the midline of the abdomen. The reference electrode is placed 10 to 15 cm to the right of the midline electrode, usually along the midclavicular line and 2 to 3 below the lowest anterior rib on the right side. The recording sites selected depend on the nature of the EGG signal desired. For example, desirable EGG signals have the largest possible amplitude, minimal artifact from ECG, respiration, and subject movement. From our experience, the electrode locations just described provide the largest possible amplitude and least artifact in EGGs from most patients. The exact placement of the electrodes is not important if the frequency of the EGG signal is what is of interest. For a discussion of the advantages and disadvantages of different electrode placements for EGG recording, see Smout et al.[2] and Mirizzi and Scafoglieri.[4]

We have sometimes recorded from two or three abdominal sites simultaneously and chosen the more artifact-free EGG signal for analysis and interpretation[5]. Chen and colleagues[6] have recorded multichannel EGGs, using four active electrodes and a common reference electrode, and reported detecting gastric slow wave propagation and quantifying the degree of slow wave coupling in normal controls and in patient groups such as individuals with systemic sclerosis.[7] The single-channel EGG recording is sufficient for diagnosing clinical gastric dysrhythmias in patients, as described in later chapters.

The EGG can be recorded from the patient's wrists, but the amplitude will be low compared with recordings from the abdomen because electrodes located on wrists are far from the source of the signal, that is, the gastric pacemaker in the corpus antrum.[8] On the other hand, wrist electrodes are recommended when recording from obese patients, to minimize the fat layer under the electrodes, which acts as an insulator and decreases the amplitude of the EGG signal. The patient's girth may also affect the amplitude of the EGG signal.

Surface Electrodes

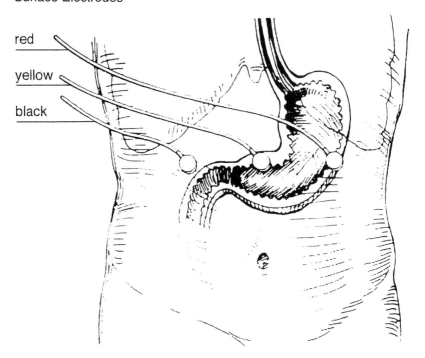

Figure 4.1. Position of electrodes on the surface of the epigastrium for recording a single-channel electrogastrogram (EGG). Electrodes labelled red and yellow are the active electrodes. Electrode red is placed 2 to 3 cm below the subject's rib cage on the left side, and electrode yellow is placed in the midline equidistant from xiphoid notch and umbilicus. The reference electrode (black) is placed on the patient's right side at least 3 cm below the right costal margin.

Procedure

Patients should be instructed on what and when to eat before an EGG recording session because the contents of the stomach affect ongoing gastric neuromuscular activity and hence EGG activity. For our research studies, subjects are instructed to fast for at least 4 hours before the experimental session. For our clinical studies, patients fast after midnight and then ingest a 200-Kcal breakfast of two pieces of toast and 4 oz. of apple juice 2 hours before the EGG test. By controlling the pretest meal, a more standardized baseline EGG is obtained before provocative testing.[9,10]

Before placement of the electrodes, the patient's skin must be prepared by shaving excess hair, gently abrading the skin, and cleaning the area with alcohol to lower electrical resistance and achieve an optimal electrode–skin interface. This is a very important part of the EGG recording procedure. If the electrical resistance between the electrode and skin is high, then the EGG signal amplitude is decreased and artifacts may increase in the signal.

The best EGG recordings are obtained if the patient reclines about 30 to 45 degrees in a comfortable chair. The patient should be instructed to minimize talking and movement during EGG recording to prevent movement artifacts. If possible, the patient should be in a quiet room separated by some distance from the person conducting the testing. Loud noises, crying children, and other stimuli that might disturb the patient and the EGG recording should be avoided. If ambulatory EGG records are desired, then Fetrodes (UFI) should be used. Fetrodes are miniature preamplifiers that are attached to the electrodes and reduce movement artifacts.

How to Minimize and Identify Artifacts

Movement of the Limbs and Body

Movement of limbs or body may physically disturb the electrode–skin interface and create movement artifacts in the EGG signal. To minimize movement artifact, follow the electrode application procedure described earlier and have patients recline comfortably as opposed to sitting upright. This position also allows the electrodes to rest on flat abdominal surfaces, not in fatty folds. Patients should also loosen their clothing so that neither a tight waistband nor a belt touches the electrodes. Also, patients should be cautioned to avoid touching the electrodes during recordings. These movements may result in a quick large-amplitude off-scale deflection of the EGG signal as shown in Figure 4.2. The length of time that the signal remains off scale depends on the amplifier used in the recording system.

Talking

Talking softly should not cause artifacts in the EGG. However, if talking is accompanied by gesturing or disturbance in normal breathing (e.g., deep breath, sigh, or cough), then artifacts in the EGG may occur. For this reason, talking by the patient during EGG recording should be kept at a minimum.

Identifying Artifacts in the Electrogastrographic Signal

Electrode and Other Electrical Failures

Figure 4.3 shows a normal 3-cpm EGG signal that suddenly becomes a flat line. This can happen if one of the active electrodes loosens or is dislodged from the skin or if there is a loss of power to or a short in the amplifier. This "flat line" artifact that occurred abruptly should not be confused with the flatline EGG signal shown in Figure 4.4. This two-channel EGG shows very little cyclic activity, but this healthy subject had not eaten for many hours and, therefore, very little organized or high-amplitude EGG activity is expected.

Respiratory Artifacts

In some cases a strong but normal respiratory signal dominates the EGG. It is not possible to filter out all respiratory signals because the frequency of respiration is close to the duodenal frequency (12–14 cpm) in some people. The extent to which respiration signals are seen in an EGG recording depends in part on the proximity of the diaphragm and stomach to the active EGG electrodes. The patient's position or posture and placement of the electrodes too close to the ribs are factors. In some cases, the patient's stomach

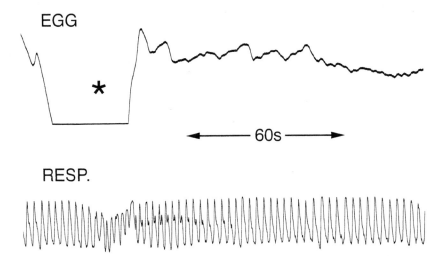

Figure 4.2. Electrogastrogram (EGG) recording showing a motion artifact (*). Note that at the point where the EGG tracing went off scale, the patient's breathing (RESP) also became irregular. Movement artifacts in the EGG must be identified and excluded from visual and computer analyses. RESP, respiration signal.

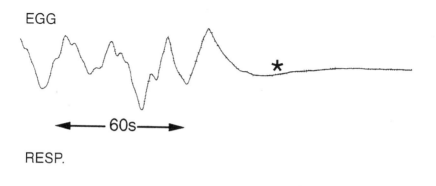

Figure 4.3. An electrogastrogram (EGG) recording that suddenly shifted from 3 cpm to flat line (*) because of an interruption in the electrical circuit. The most common cause of such an artifact would be an active electrode becoming loose or dislodged from the skin. RESP, respiration signal.

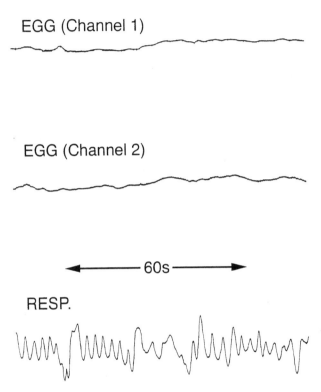

EGG (Channel 1)

EGG (Channel 2)

◄——— 60s ———►

RESP.

Figure 4.4. Two channels of electrogastrogram (EGG) recorded simultaneously from a patient who had fasted for 12 hours. There is some undulation in the EGG signal but very little cyclical EGG activity, as would be expected from a person who had not eaten for many hours. Note that the EGG recordings are not a flat line, however, as seen in the artifact in Figure 4.3. Changes in respiration rate do not affect the EGG signal in this patient. RESP, respiration signal.

moves with each breath, producing the respiratory frequencies in the EGG tracing. The only way to know if a series of waves in the EGG recording is being generated by the stomach or by respiration is to record respiration separately and compare the two records. For example, after the water load test, a considerable amount of tachygastria (7 cpm) may be seen in the EGG signal, as shown in Figure 4.5. However, the separate recording of respiration (Figure 4.5, insert B) showed that the apparent tachygastria was an artifact caused by respiration that occurred at the identical rate of 7 breaths per minute.

Harmonics

If the shape of the EGG signal departs greatly from a smooth sinusoidal curve and has sharp or flat contours, then the fast-fourier transform (FFT) decomposes the signal into subcomponents that are multiples of the basic or primary frequency in the EGG signal. These subcomponent frequencies are called *harmonics*. Figure 4.6 (top) shows an example of an EGG with nonsinusoidal waves (note the flat tops of the 3-cpm EGG waves). Figure 4.6 (bottom) shows the running spectral analysis (RSA) of this EGG recording. The RSA shows that the greatest power is at 3 cpm, but there also are peaks with progressively less power at 6 cpm and even less power at 9 cpm. The frequencies and power at 6 and 9 cpm are harmonics and are not tachygastrias. Harmonics can be identified easily because they are multiples of the primary EGG frequency and always have less power than the primary frequency, as shown in Figure 4.6. Furthermore, inspection of the raw EGG signal shows 3-cpm waves and fails to show waves at 6 cpm or 9 cpm.

Summary

Recording the EGG is relatively simple with the hardware and software now available specifically for that purpose. However, one must apply the electrodes properly and inspect the raw EGG signal carefully to identify quality EGG signals. Any artifacts in the EGG signal should be identified and excluded from visual or computer analysis.

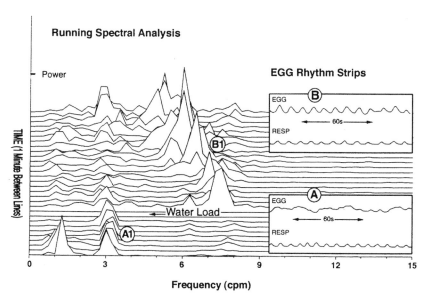

Figure 4.5. Electrogastrogram (EGG) rhythm strips and running spectral analysis (RSA) before and after the water load test in a patient with unexplained nausea. The baseline EGG signal (A) shows 3-cpm waves, and in the RSA, 3-cpm peaks are seen (A1). After the water load, there appeared to be a considerable amount of tachygastria (e.g., 7 cpm) in the RSA (B1). However, in the actual recording of the EGG rhythm strip (B), the apparent 7-cpm tachygastria is actually caused by respirations that were occurring at 7 breaths per minute. Respirations (Resp) are shown with the EGG rhythm strip.

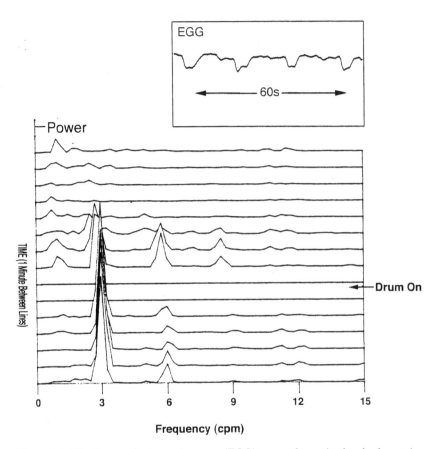

Figure 4.6. The 3-cpm electrogastrogram (EGG) waves shown in the rhythm strip at the top of the figure have flat tops and are not sinusoid-type waves. The running spectral analysis (RSA) of this EGG signal before and after "Drum On" shows high-power peaks at 3 cpm and lower-power harmonic peaks at 6 and even lower-power peaks at 9 cpm. Harmonics in the RSA are expected if the raw EGG signal has flat or pointy tops, and thus varies from the sinusoidal shape. (See Fig. 3.15 for an example of EGG signals with more pointed peaks and the associated harmonics in the RSA.) The two flat lines in the RSA at "Drum On," indicates the time at which drum rotation began for this motion sickness study.

References

1. Koch KL, Stern RM: Electrogastrographic data acquisition and analysis: the Penn State experience. In: Chen JZ, McCallum RW, eds. *Electrogastrography*, New York: Raven Press;1994:31–44.

2. Smout AJPM, Jebbink HJA, Samsom M: Acquisition and analysis of electrogastrographic data: the Dutch experience. In: Chen JZ, McCallum RW, eds. *Electrogastrography*, New York: Raven Press;1994:3–30.

3. Stern RM, Koch KL, Muth ER: Gastrointestinal system. In: Cacioppo JT, Tassinary LG, Berntson GG, eds. *Handbook of Psychophysiology*, 2nd ed. New York: Cambridge University Press; 2000:294–314.

4. Mirizzi N, Scafoglieri U: Optimal directions of the electrogastrographic signal in man. *Med Biol Eng Comp* 1983;21:385–389.

5. Stern RM, Koch KL, Leibowitz HW, et al: Tachygastria and motion sickness. *Aviat Space Environ Med* 1985;56:1074–1077.

6. Chen JDZ, Zou XP, Lin XM, et al: Detection of gastric slow wave propagation from the cutaneous electrogastrogram. *Am J Physiol* 1996;277: G424–G430.

7. McNearney T, Lin X, Shrestha J, et al: Characterization of gastric myoelectrical rhythms in patients with systemic sclerosis using multichannel surface electrogastrography. *Dig Dis Sci* 2002;47:690–698.

8. Stern RM, Stacher G. Recording the electrogastrogram from parts of the body surface distant from the stomach. *Psychophysiology* 1982;19:350.

9. Koch KL, Hong S-P, Xu L: Reproducibility of gastric myoelectrical activity and the water load test in patients with dysmotility-like dyspepsia symptoms and in control subjects. *J Clin Gastroenterol* 2000;31(2):125–129.

10. Koch KL. Electrogastrography. In: Schuster M, Crowel M, Koch KL, eds. *Atlas of Gastrointestinal Motility*. Hamilton, Ontario, Canada: BC Decker; 2002.

5

Analysis of the Electrogastrogram

*T*he analysis of electrogastrogram (EGG) recordings involves an initial visual inspection of the signal to assess the quality of the signal, identification of artifacts, and selection of the minutes of EGG signal to analyze visually and by computer. This chapter discusses an approach to analyses of the EGG for clinical and research studies.

Visual Analysis of Electrogastrographic Signal

All raw EGG recordings must be visually inspected to identify 3–cycles per minute (cpm) signals, gastric dysrhythmias, and any artifacts in the signal. Certain characteristics of the EGG can be determined and qualitative judgments can be made on the basis of visual inspection of an EGG record. Artifact-free minutes of the EGG signal must be selected for use in analyses that are generated by computer programs.

When inspecting the EGG recording, there are several important questions to ask:

1. Is the baseline EGG recording rhythmic or dysrhythmic?
2. Are bradygastria, normal, or tachygastria frequencies identifible?
3. Is the amplitude of the EGG signal low, medium, or high?
4. After a provocative stimulus, does the EGG signal become more or less rhythmic? For example, Figure 5.1 shows a normal 3-cpm EGG signal that shifts to a tachygastria as the subject experienced nausea in a rotating optokinetic drum.[1] Clinically relevant gastric dysrhythmias are persistent and last at least 3 to 5 minutes, usually much longer.
5. Is there a normal increase in the amplitude of the EGG after eating? Figure 5.2 shows an EGG recorded from a healthy subject before and after eating a test breakfast meal. Note the obvious increase in EGG amplitude at 3 cpm after the ingestion of food.
6. Are there artifacts in the EGG signal associated with movements of limbs or body or changes in respiration? Portions of the EGG recording with artifacts must be identified and not submitted for computer analysis; otherwise, erroneous data quantitative data will be generated.

Thus, frequency and amplitude of the raw EGG signal during baseline and in response to the test stimulus should be first assessed visually.[2,3] The visual inspection of the EGG record determines the general quality of the EGG signal and the presence of any artifacts. In the examples in this and other chapters, actual EGG tracings are shown, as well as running spectral analyses (RSAs) of EGG recordings.

Computer Analysis of the Electrogastrographic Signal

There are three steps involved in the computer-aided quantitative analysis of the EGG[2]:

1. The EGG recording is filtered digitally to remove unwanted frequencies such as 0.5-cpm ultraslow drift and respiratory and cardiac rhythms.

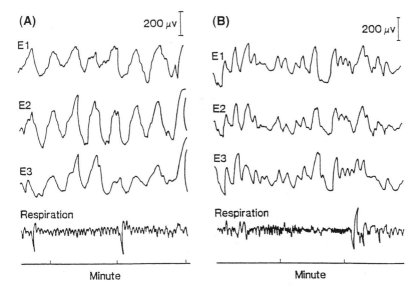

Figure 5.1. Electrogastrogram (EGG) activity recorded from three channels (E1–E3) before rotation of a optokinetic drum used to evoke motion sickness and nausea symptoms. EGG signals before drum rotation (A) show a clear, normal 3-cpm pattern in all channels. EGG signals from the same subject during rotation of the optokinetic drum are shown (B). Note the presence of 6- to 7-cpm tachygastria in all channels. The tachygastria began at minute 4 of drum rotation, and the subject reported nausea at minute 6. The subject requested termination of the session at minute 11 of drum rotation. (Reprinted with permission from Stern et al., 1985).

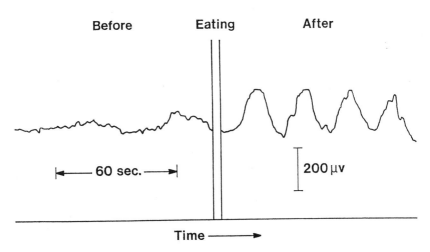

Figure 5.2. Electrogastrogram (EGG) signal recorded from a healthy subject before and after eating a breakfast of juice, cold cereal with milk, two pieces of toast with butter and jam, and coffee. The EGG signal recorded *before* eating shows a low-amplitude 1- to 2-cpm EGG signal. The EGG signal on the right was recorded from the same subject 5 minutes *after* the breakfast. Note the normal 3-cpm EGG activity after ingestion of the meal.

2. A spectral analysis is performed on the selected artifact-free minutes of EGG signal to quantify the different frequencies of interest in the signal.
3. Specific EGG parameters, such as percentage distribution of EGG power, are calculated.

Filters and the Electrogastrographic Signal

Conventional bandpass filters. To record a high-quality EGG, myoelectrical activity that occurs at lower or higher frequencies must be filtered out.[2,3] These filters reduce baseline drift and eliminate most respiratory and cardiac rhythms. Using a 0.016-Hz (≈1-cpm) high-pass filter and a 0.25-Hz (15-cpm) low-pass filter, a bandpass from 1 to 15 cpm is achieved. The combination of these two filters is considered a *bandpass filter.* The bandpass filter just described allows only frequencies between 1 and 15 cpm to reach the amplifier. The frequencies of interest from the stomach and duodenum are within the range of 1 to 15 cpm: bradygastria (1–2.5 cpm), normal range (2.5–3.75 cpm), tachygastria (3.75–10.0 cpm), and duodenal/respiration (10–15 cpm).

A bandpass filter is the most straightforward method of filtering unwanted frequencies, but it does affect the phase or wave form of the signal. Some motion artifacts and respiration signals (e.g., respiration rates of 12 per minute) may not be filtered out (see Chapter 4, Figure 4.5). The clinician can deal with these limitations of bandpass filters by minimizing patient movement and recording respiration on a separate channel.

Adaptive filtering. In adaptive filtering, a separate reference signal is used as an error signal or noise, which is subtracted from the primary signal of interest. For further discussion of adaptive filtering, see Ref. 4

Spectral Analysis of the Electrogastrographic Signal

Fourier analysis, running spectral analysis (RSA), and adaptive spectral analysis are computational methods used to determine the frequencies contained in the EGG signal.

Fourier analysis. When the EGG signal undergoes a fast-Fourier transform (FFT), the result is analogous to shining a light through a prism and seeing the many individual colors that make up the original light. Fourier was a French mathematician who suggested that any given time series can be described as a corresponding sum of sine and cosine functions. Therefore, the output of an FFT is an estimate of the power of the various frequencies that composed the original signal. Power, sometimes expressed as decibels or microvolts squared, is an index of the amplitude of the sinusoidal-shaped waves of the particular frequencies that would be required to recreate the EGG signal.

In the FFT analysis of EGG recordings, the power in the bradygastria, normal, tachygastria, and duodenal/respiration ranges is determined.[2] Figures 7.4 through 7.6 show the FFTs for 4 minutes of EGG signal in the normal, tachygastria, and bradygastria ranges. The percentage of all of the EGG power from 1 to 15 cpm in each of the four relevant frequency ranges is also expressed as the percentage distribution of EGG power. Ratios of the power can be calculated to indicate the changes within a frequency band of interest before and after a test meal or stimulus.[6] The power value itself can also be used as a quantitative measure.[4,5] As discussed later, the percentage distribution of EGG power in the four relevant frequency ranges is an ideal measure for clinical EGG studies for the following reasons: (1) All frequencies from 1 to 15 cpm are evaluated, (2) Small changes in nondominant frequencies are clinically relevant to symptoms like nausea and bloating, and (3) The percentage distribution of EGG power is ideal for comparison of individual patients with healthy volunteers.

Running Spectral Analysis (RSA)

Van der Schee, Smout, and Grashuis[5] described modifications of the spectral analysis method—the RSA—to quantify frequencies in the EGG signal. The RSA is of interest because it provides EGG frequency and power information *over time*, whereas the FFT provides only power as a function of frequency. Figure 5.3 shows FFTs of 2 minutes of EGG signal before and after a meal. Figure 5.4 shows an RSA of a 15-minute baseline EGG followed by 30 minutes of EGG signal recorded after the subject ingested 550 ml of water. In the RSA, the power of each of the four relevant frequency ranges in the EGG can be seen in the pseudo–three-dimensional (3D) plot. The clear peaks at 3 cpm in the RSA (B) correspond to the clear 3-cpm waves seen in the rhythm strip. Other examples of RSAs of EGG signals appear throughout this book.

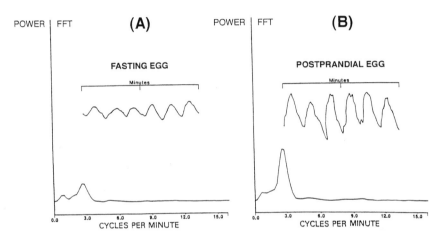

Figure 5.3. Two-minute electrogastrogram (EGG) rhythm strips and correspond-ing fast-fourier transform (FFT) recorded from a healthy subject. (*A*) The EGG recorded during fasting shows a low-amplitude 3-cpm EGG signal. The FFT plot of this signal shows a low-power peak at 3 cpm. (*B*) The postprandial EGG signal from the same subject after ingesting two pieces of toast and 8 oz. of apple juice shows an increase in amplitude in the 3-cpm EGG waves. The FFT shows a corre-sponding increase in power at 3 cpm.

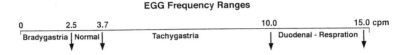

EGG Frequency Ranges

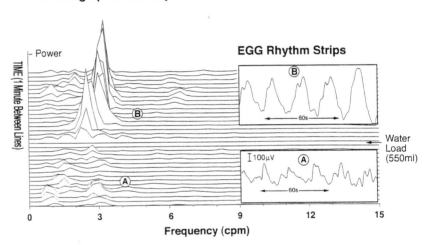

Figure 5.4. The running spectral analysis (RSA) is shown with frequency in cpm on the X-axis, time in minutes going from bottom to top on the Y-axis, and power is depicted as the peaks in the z-axis. During baseline, the subject had low-amplitude 3-cpm EGG waves (see A in EGG rhythm strip). Note the corresponding peaks at 3 cpm in the RSA (A). After 550 ml of water was ingested during the water load test, frequency decreased briefly to approximately 2-cpm, followed by clear 3-cpm peaks of increased power in the RSA (B). The EGG rhythm strip from after water ingestion (B) shows increased amplitude and regularity of 3-cpm activity. Thus, increases in the amplitude of EGG waves are reflected as increases in power in the RSA at that frequency. The frequency ranges of relevance (bradygastria, normal, tachygastria, and duodenal respiration) are shown above the RSA and are discussed further in Chapters through 6–8.

The mathematical procedures used to convert the raw EGG signal to an RSA and pseudo-3D are described later. These procedures are carried out automatically with proprietary EGG hardware and software sold by medical equipment companies, but the first step in any quantification procedure is to ensure that quality data are being analyzed.[7] Hence, time must be taken to ensure the quality of EGG recordings before computer analyses are undertaken. The amplifying and recording system should filter out signals below 1.0 cpm and above 15 cpm.[2] With these filter settings, the slow rhythms (1.0–2.5 cpm) are recorded accurately and the shifts in baseline due to direct-current potentials that are less than 0.5 cpm are eliminated. Frequencies higher than 15 cpm are filtered out to avoid contamination of the gastric signal by electrocardiographic (ECG) signals. Respiration signals can obscure the EGG when breathing rates falls near that of tachygastria (3.7–10 cpm) or duodenal slow wave frequencies (12–14 cpm). Removal of respiration signals by setting the low-pass filter at 10 cpm or less would also remove duodenal signals. Therefore, a separate respiration tracing is used to select visually and exclude minutes that contain the obvious artifacts related to respiratory rates or movement artifacts.

The EGG signal is channeled from the amplifier to an analog to digital (A/D) converter. The signal is digitized into a series of numerical values representing discrete voltage levels of the raw EGG signal. Analog to digital conversion devices typically allow a wide range of sampling rates. For more than 20 years, we have used 4.267 Hz for our sampling rate because it yields 256 data points per minute, and 256 is a power of 2 (2^8), a requirement for the spectral analysis we use. Regardless of the analysis method used, we recommend a sampling rate of at least 1 Hz to eliminate the potential for aliasing. *Aliasing* refers to the process whereby unwanted high-frequency components, such as the ECG, appear under the alias of the wanted low-frequency signal, in this case, the EGG. Although the EGG signal is subjected to a high-frequency filter with a low cutoff of 15 cpm, some ECG frequencies may still be present but attenuated by the filter. If aliasing is not eliminated before computer analysis, some ECG power is erroneously added to the EGG power. This is referred to as *leakage*. A high sampling rate for EGG recording, such as 4.267 Hz, allows complete resolution of all potential frequencies in the EGG signal and thus prevents aliasing.

Once the entire EGG recording has been digitized, the data must be preprocessed to meet the assumptions of FFT analysis. Because the normal 3-cpm frequency in the EGG is a relatively slow frequency, we recommend the analysis of at least 4 minutes of EGG data. The data are "centered" for spectral analysis around a mean of zero. This is accomplished by subtracting the mean of the data segment from each individual data point. In addition, the EGG is likely to contain some ultraslow components (<0.5 cpm) that reflect drifting baseline as described earlier. These ultraslow components may not be completely filtered out by the bandpass filter. Such extremely low-frequency shifts and simple linear trends should be removed. A high-pass digital filter that attenuates frequencies below 0.01 Hz (0.6 cpm) accomplishes the removal of ultraslow-frequency components in the digitized EGG data. One can also remove simple linear trends by fitting a least-squares regression line and subtracting it from the data segment. Thus, the analog EGG signal is converted to a digital series of values and placed in a file that is subjected to various quantitative analyses.

Figure 5.5 shows the steps involved in the processing of the digitized EGG file. A raw EGG segment of 4 minutes duration is shown in Figure 5.5A. This data segment shows an obvious upward drift in the baseline during the 240-second recording. The segment was first zero-centered, and the baseline shift was removed using a high-pass filter (Fig. 5.5B). Next, this segment of EGG signal was "windowed" to reduce leakage. *Windowing* is the application of a weighting function that tapers the beginning and end of the data segment to zero. Thus, the middle of the segment is unaltered, or multiplied by a weight of one, whereas the ends are multiplied by weights gradually approaching zero (Fig. 5.5C). This is necessary because when a signal abruptly terminates at the beginning or end of a recording or segment, there is leakage in the power spectrum. Note that the windowing procedure shown in Figure 5.5C results in a gradual tapering of the signal to zero at each end of the 4-minute EGG segment. This procedure greatly reduces leakage. The window applied in this example is a Hamming window. However, many other windows may be chosen depending on the characteristics of the signal (see Chen[4] for a discussion of various windowing techniques for use with EGG). In general, windows such as the Hamming, Hanning, and Tukey-Blackman provide comparable results when used with EGG.

After the preprocessing steps for the EGG signal are completed, the data undergo the FFT. The power at each frequency in the EGG signal is obtained. The frequencies present in a 4-minute EGG signal, as determined by the FFT, are shown in (Fig. 5.5D). Note that the

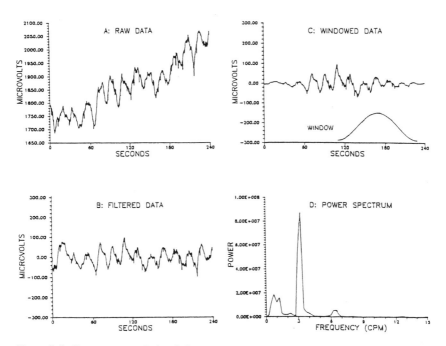

Figure 5.5. Computer analysis of electrogastrogram (EGG) signals. (*A*) Raw data. The raw EGG signal shows considerable drift in baseline from 60 to 240 seconds compared with 0- to 60-second period. (*B*) Filtered data. The same EGG signal is shown after zero-centering and removal of baseline drift with a high-pass filter. (*C*) Windowed data. The same EGG signal is shown after a Hamming window was applied. The Hamming window is shown below the windowed EGG data. The shape of the Hamming window indicates that data in the middle of the EGG data segment were weighted most heavily and the weighting approached zero at the two ends of the EGG data segment. (*D*) Power spectrum. Fast Fourier transform (FFT) of the windowed EGG data from (*C*) is shown. Note the prominent peak at 3 cpm and the power at this frequency. Much less power is associated with the peaks at 1 and 6 cpm. (Reprinted with permission from Stern et al., 2000.)

frequency with greatest power occurred at 3 cpm. Peaks with little power are seen at 1 and 6 cpm.

Consecutive 4-minute EGG data "segments" are overlapped to produce an RSA that displays frequency and power over time. We use a 75% overlap in both clinical and research recordings. In other words, "segment" 1 contains minutes 1 to 4 of EGG data, segment 2 includes minutes 2 to 5, segment 3 includes minutes 3 to 6, and so on. Thus, 1 minute of a new EGG signal (e.g. minute 6) is added to the previous 3 minutes of EGG signal (minutes 3, 4, and 5), thus accomplishing the 75% overlap. An FFT is then performed on each of the overlapped 4-minute EGG data segments. These overlapping power spectra are plotted in a pseudo-3D fashion to determine changes in power at various frequencies over time. The calculation of specific EGG parameters is discussed later in this chapter.

RSAs provide an informative picture of EGG frequency and power changes over time. EGG frequency changes of 60 seconds or longer usually appear as a concordant change at that frequency in the RSA.[5] It should be noted that frequency changes lasting less than 60 seconds may not be detected. Adaptive spectral analysis methods may be used if frequency changes less than 60 seconds are of interest.[8,9] For clinical EGG uses, changes in the EGG frequencies lasting longer than 60 seconds are considered relevant to establishing the diagnosis of tachygastria or bradygastria and are easily seen in the raw EGG recording. Furthermore, dysrhythmias with a duraction of longer than 60 seconds are considered clinically significant and are easily seen in the raw EGG recording and in the RSA.[5]

FFT and RSA are particularly useful when the EGG signal contains a significant amount of cyclic activity. When bursts of tachygastria are seen during motion sickness or in patients in response to the water load test, they are typically 1 or more minutes in duration and are seen clearly in running spectral plots of 4-minute epochs.[10] Other methods of analysis for quantification of signals lasting several seconds are available; see, for example, Hölzl et al.[11] for a discussion of zoom FFTs and Lin and Chen[8] for a discussion of adaptive spectral analysis.

Adaptive spectral analysis. Adaptive spectral analysis of the EGG signal is based on autoregressive moving average modeling.[8] Figure 5.6 shows 10 minutes of raw EGG data and the corresponding RSA plot calculated by the adaptive spectral analysis method. As can be seen, the EGG signal contains both a 3-cpm component and another signal, perhaps

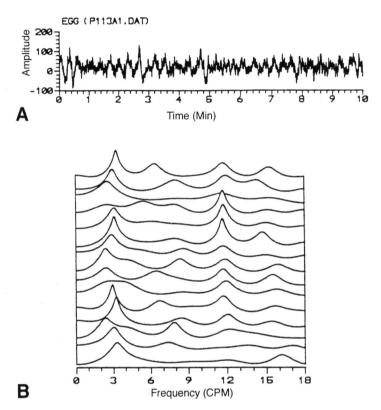

Figure 5.6. Electrogastrogram (EGG) recording (*A*) and spectral analysis from the adaptive method (*B*). The EGG recording (*A*) shows 10 minutes of signal and 3-cpm waves are present. The frequency analysis (*B*) indicates peaks at 3 cpm and regular peaks at 12 cpm. Each line represents the frequencies in 2 minutes of the EGG signal. (Reprinted with permission of Raven Press[8].)

from respiration, at 12 cpm. The running spectral plot shows the separation of two primary frequencies in the signal as two peaks of power, one at 3 cpm and the other at 12 cpm. Adaptive spectral analysis has been used in research settings where detection of brief periods of dysrhythmia in the EGG signal (<60 seconds) are desired. FFT or adaptive analysis may be used if temporal resolution for 1 minute of EGG signal is needed. A disadvantage of adaptive spectral analysis in clinical EGG testing is that it may fail to accurately present the relative amplitude of the different frequencies that compose a typical EGG signal.[8]

Specific Electrogastrographic Parameters

1. *Percentage distribution of electrogastrographic power in the four frequency bands of interest.* The percentage distribution of EGG power in the four relevant frequency bands is the measure that the authors have found most useful in more than 20 years of experience in recording and analyzing EGGs in studies involving patients and healthy research participants.[2,3,12] The percentage distribution of total EGG power is calculated for each of the frequency bands of interest: bradygastria, normal 3 cpm, tachygastria, and duodenal/respiration. The power estimates for a given frequency range (e.g., the 1–2.5 bradygastria range) are obtained from the spectral analysis. The sum of the bradygastria power for a given time period is divided by the power for the entire frequency range (1–15 cpm) for the same time period and multiplied by 100%. Thus, the percentage distribution of *all* of the power from 1 to 15 cpm is determined for each of the four relevant frequency ranges: bradygastria, normal, tachygastria, and duodenal/respiration. The percentage of EGG power in the different frequency bands is altered by provocative stimuli such as the water load test or a caloric meal or drug therapy. This measure should not be confused with percentage of *time* with the dominant frequency in the normal (or other) frequency bands, which is described next.

2. *Percentage of time with the dominant frequency in the normal (or other) frequency band.* This measure calculates the percentage of time (within a defined period) that the dominant EGG frequency (the specific frequency with the greatest power as determined by computer analysis) lies within a certain range of frequencies, such as 2–4 cpm.[13] An adaptive filter analysis of the EGG is first computed

using 1 or 2 minutes of EGG data to construct each power spectra. A spectrum is considered normal if the dominant (highest) peak lies in the 2- to 4-cpm range. The percentage of time that the highest peak is in the 2- to 4-cpm range is determined visually. Thus, if eight 1-minute spectra had the highest peak in the 2- to 4-cpm range in a 10-minute period, then the percentage of time the dominant frequency was in the normal range would be 80%.

A limitation of this measure is that it ignores much of the data present in the EGG signal and focuses solely on the time that the dominant frequency is or is not within the frequency range of interest.

For example, a 2-minute EGG signal with six 20-second sine waves or a 2-minute EGG signal with one large 20-second sine wave and a variety of other low-amplitude waves spread out in frequencies other than 2 to 4 cpm would be labeled normal. This is why the percentage of time measure produces higher percentages of normal activity compared with the percentage distribution of EGG power, the technique described previously. Recall that the percentage distribution of EGG power compares the 3-cpm activity present in the EGG signal with the activity in all frequencies from 1 to 15 cpm for a given period of time. Compared with that method, the percentage of time with the dominant frequency in the normal-frequency band includes only a small, select portion of the total EGG data. Therefore, investigators who use this measure may arrive at erroneous conclusions about the effects of a drug or other therapy on EGG because of the selective nature of the data that are included in this measure. In addition, the percentage of time with the dominant frequency in the normal range is usually derived from an adaptative spectral analysis, not a Fourier spectral analysis, and therefore does not always accurately present the relative amplitude of the different frequencies that compose the EGG signal.

3. *Power ratio.* The EGG activity in the frequency band of interest after a test or therapy is compared with EGG activity in that same frequency band during the baseline period. For example, a clinician might calculate the ratio of power in the normal range before and after treatment with a particular drug used to reduce nausea and use the ratio as a measure of improvement. However, an increase in EGG activity in all frequency

bands may occur and would make interpretation of the specific ratio difficult.

4. *Dominant frequency and stability of the dominant frequency.* The dominant frequency is determined visually by identifying the frequency with the greatest power in the FTT or RSA during a specific time period. Frequencies can change even in healthy subjects. Note that a frequency dip to 1 to 2 cpm occurs briefly after a meal (see Fig. 5.3B). Smout, Jebbink, and Samsom[14] calculated various measures of stability of the dominant frequency and concluded that there is little evidence that either dominant frequency or the stability of the dominant frequency is physiologically related to gastric function.

Analysis of clinical EGG recordings is based on the recording of high-quality EGG signals, review of the signal to identify any artifacts, and use of validated software for quantitative analysis of the EGG signal.[15] The computer analysis provides quantification of the frequencies that are seen in the EGG signal, as reviewed in the next chapters. With use of these techniques, EGG recordings and analyses can be confidently interpreted for research and clinical uses.

References

1. Stern RM, Koch RM, Leibowitz HW, et al: Tachygastria and motion sickness. *Aviat Space Envir Med* 1985;56:1074–1077.
2. Stern RM, Koch KL, Muth ER: The gastrointestinal system. In: Cacioppo JT, Tessinary LG, Berntson GG, eds. *Handbook of Psychophysiology*, 2nd ed. Cambridge: Cambridge University Press; 2000: 294–314.
3. Koch KL: Electrogastrography. In: Schuster M, Crowel M, Koch KL, eds. *Atlas of Gastrointestinal Motility.* Hamilton, Ontario, Canada, BC Decker; 2002.
4. Chen J: Signal processing and analysis. *Neurogastroenterology* 2000;3: 104–112.
5. Van der Schee EJ, Smout AJPM, Grashuis JL: Application of running spectrum analysis to electrogastrographic signals recorded from dog and man. In M. Wienbeck (Ed.), *Motility Digestive Tract.* New York: Raven Press; 1982:241–250.
6. Geldof H, van der Schee EJ, van Blankenstein M, et al: Electrogastrographic study of gastric myoelectrical activity in patients with unexplained nausea and vomiting. *Gut* 1986;27:799–808.
7. Kingma YJ: The electrogastrogram and its analysis. *Crit Rev Biomed Eng* 1989; 17:105–132.

8. Lin Z, Chen JZ: Comparison of three spectral analysis methods. In Chen JZ, McCallum RW, eds., *Electrogastrography*. New York: Raven Press; 1994:75–102.

9. Chen JD, Stewart WR, McCallum RW. Spectral analysis of episodic rhythmic variations in the cutaneous electrogastrogram. *IEEE Trans Biomed Eng* 1993;40:128–135.

10. Stern RM, Koch KL, Stewart WR, et al: Spectral analysis of tachygastria recorded during motion sickness. *Gastroenterology* 1987;92:92–97.

11. Hölzl R, Löffler K, Müller GM: On conjoint gastrography or what the surface gastrogram shows. In Stern RM, Koch KL, eds. *Electrogastrography*. New York: Praeger; 1985:89–115.

12. Koch KL, Hong S-P, Xu L: Reproducibility of gastric myoelectrical activity and the water load test in patients with dysmotility-like dyspepsia symptoms and in control subjects. *J Clin Gastroenterol* 2000;31:125–129.

13. Chen JZ, McCallum RW: Electrogastrographic parameters and their clinical significance. In Chen JZ, McCallum RW, eds. *Electrogastrography*. New York: Raven Press; 1994:45–74.

14. Smout AJPM, Jebbink HJA, Samsom M: Acquisition and analysis of electrogastrographic data: the Dutch experience. In Chen JZ, McCallum RW, eds. *Electrogastrography*. New York: Raven Press; 1994:3–30.

15. VerHagen MAMT, van Schelven CJ, Samsom M, et al: Pitfalls in the analysis of electrogastrographic recordings. *Gastroenterology* 1999;117: 453–460.

6

Clinical Applications of Electrogastrography

*E*lectrogastrography methods have been used in many clinical studies over the past 80 years. In 1922, Alvarez[1] predicted that electrical abnormalities of the stomach may be related to gastrointestinal (GI) symptoms and abnormal gastric function. In 1980, antral dysrhythmias were recorded with mucosal electrodes in a series of patients with unexplained nausea and vomiting.[2,3] These gastric dysrhythmias were 6– to 7–cycles per minute (cpm) tachygastrias, but there were also very irregular rhythms that changed from bradygastria to tachygastria (mixed dysrhythmias or tachyarrhythmias). Bradygastrias also were recorded in patients with unexplained nausea and vomiting.[2-6] Further studies showed a relationship between the presence of nausea and gastric dysrhythmias during motion sickness,[7,8] in nausea and vomiting of pregnancy,[9,10] and in patients with idiopathic and diabetic gastroparesis.[11-14] Infusion of a variety of drugs and physical distention of the antrum also induced gastric dysrhythmias and symptoms of nausea.[15-21] Ischemic gastroparesis with gastric dysrhythmias due to chronic mesenteric ischemia is an unusual cause of chronic nausea and vomiting.[22,23] Ischemic gastroparesis is important to recognize because after revascularization the symptoms resolved, the gastric dysrhythmias were eradicated and normal 3-cpm EGG activity and normal gastric emptying were restored. Thus, gastric dysrhythmias are found in many disorders in which nausea and vomiting are prominent symptoms. Clinical conditions associated with gastric dysrhythmias were reviewed.[24] Finally, a variety of drugs and nondrug therapies convert gastric dysrhythmias to normal 3-cpm gastric myoelectrical rhythms and the correction of the gastric dysrhythmia correlates with improvement in symptoms.[12,25–30]

Taken together, these findings indicate that gastric dysrhythmias are objective, pathophysiological events related to the upper GI symptoms, especially nausea and dysmotility-like functional dyspepsia symptoms such as early satiety, fullness, and vomiting.[26,27,31,32] The recording of gastric dysrhythmias is an important tool for the clinician when patients have symptoms that suggest gastric dysfunction such as unexplained nausea, bloating, postprandial fullness, and early satiety. On the other hand, these upper GI symptoms are nonspecific, and diseases or disorders of other organ systems such as esophagus, gallbladder, small bowel, colon, and non-GI diseases must be considered.[33,34]

The focus of this chapter is neuromuscular disorders of the stomach and the use of electrogastrography in evaluating patients with unexplained nausea and dyspepsia symptoms. Structural, infectious, and biochemical disorders that may cause these symptoms must be excluded. Gastric neuromuscular disorders such as gastric dysrhythmias and gastroparesis and disorders of electrical and contractile activity of the stomach are then considered.

An Approach to the Patient with Dyspepsia Symptoms

Dyspepsia means "bad digestion." Thus, dyspepsia symptoms are usually worse after the patient ingests food. The symptoms include postprandial nausea, early satiety, prolonged fullness, vague epigastric discomfort (not pain), and vomiting.[33] These are indeed nonspecific symptoms and may be caused by a variety of diseases and disorders (Table 6.1). The symptoms are also approached differently depending on where the patient first presents for evaluation. If the patient is first evaluated by a primary care physician, then an empiric trial of an acid suppression or a promotility agent may be given if there are

Table 6.1. Differential Diagnosis of Nausea and Vomiting

1. Mechanical obstruction
   Pylorus, duodenum, small intestine, colon

2. Postgastric surgery
   Vagotomy/antrectomy, Roux-en-Y, funduplication

3. Metabolic/endocrine disorders
   Diabetic mellitus, hypothyroidism, hyperthyroidism, adrenal insufficiency

4. Medications
   Anticholinergics, narcotics, L-dopa, progesterone, calcium channel blockers

5. Chronic mesenteric ischemia

6. Psychogenic disorders
   Anorexia nervosa, bulimia

7. Smooth muscle disorders
   Hollow viscus myopathy, scleroderma muscular dystrophy

8. Neuropathic disorders
   Hollow viscus neuropathy, Parkinson's, paraneoplastic syndrome,
   Shy-Drager

9. Postviral gastroparesis

10. Idiopathic gastroparesis with or without gastric dysrhythmias

no alarm symptoms present. If alarm symptoms such as severe abdominal pain, hematemesis, weight loss, age of greater than 50 years, or other known and relevant diseases and disorders are present, then a diagnostic evaluation should begin.[33,35]

If the patient presents to a gastroenterologist, then frequently empiric trials of drugs have already been given. An upper GI series and a computed tomography scan often have been performed, and the results are normal. Figure 6.1 outlines an approach for these patients that incorporates the primary care physician's and the gastroenterologist's evaluation of the patient with common dyspepsia symptoms. First, if empiric therapy fails to improve these symptoms, then a straightforward evaluation of the symptoms includes routine blood tests, an upper endoscopy, and an abdominal ultrasonogram. The blood tests rule out anemia, electrolyte disturbances, abnormal liver function, and hypothyroidism. An upper endoscopy is performed to diagnose mucosal diseases of the esophagus, stomach, and

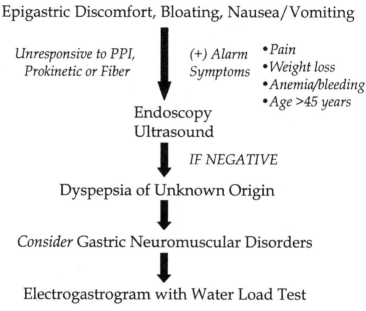

Epigastric Discomfort, Bloating, Nausea/Vomiting

Unresponsive to PPI,
Prokinetic or Fiber

(+) Alarm
Symptoms

- *Pain*
- *Weight loss*
- *Anemia/bleeding*
- *Age >45 years*

Endoscopy
Ultrasound

IF NEGATIVE

Dyspepsia of Unknown Origin

Consider Gastric Neuromuscular Disorders

Electrogastrogram with Water Load Test

Figure 6.1. Algorithm for evaluating patients with uninvestigated epigastric discomfort, bloating, nausea, and vomiting (dyspepsia symptoms). If alarm symptoms are present, then the evaluation should proceed with endoscopy and ultrasound of the gallbladder and pancreas to rule out mucosal or structural diseases and disorders. If the cause of dyspepsia symptoms remains unknown, then gastric neuromuscular disorders should be considered. An electrogastrogram and gastric emptying study are non-invasive measures of gastric electrical and contractile activity.

duodenum. Esophagitis, gastritis, or duodenitis or pyloric obstruction may be detected. An abdominal ultrasonogram may reveal chronic cholecystitis or cholelithiasis and exclude major structural disease of the pancreas. If any specific relevant mucosal or structural abnormalities are found, then they can be treated specifically.

However, almost 50% of the patients who are referred to gastroenterologists with these symptoms have normal upper endoscopy studies.[36,37] These patients also have normal abdominal ultrasound examinations and normal blood tests. Their symptoms can be categorized as dysmotility-like functional dyspepsia or ulcer-like functional dyspepsia[33] (Table 6.2). Gastric neuromuscular dysfunction may be the cause of these symptoms. EGG and gastric emptying tests

Table 6.2. Symptoms of Functional Dyspepsia

Symptom	Definition
Ulcer-like Functional Dyspepsia	
Pain centered in the upper abdomen	*Pain* refers to a subjective, unpleasant sensation; some patients may feel that tissue damage is occurring. Other symptoms may be extremely bothersome without being interpreted by the patient as pain. By questioning the patient, pain should be distinguished from discomfort.
Dysmotility-like Functional Dyspepsia	
Discomfort centered in the upper abdomen	A subjective, unpleasant sensation or feeling that is not interpreted as pain according to the patient and that, if fully assessed, can include any of the symptoms below.
Early satiety	A feeling that the stomach is overfilled soon after starting to eat, out of proportion to the size of the meal being eaten, so that the meal cannot be finished.
Fullness	An unpleasant sensation like the persistence of food in the stomach; this may or may not occur *postprandially* (slow digestion).
Bloating in the upper abdomen	A tightness located in the upper abdomen; it should be distinguished from visible abdominal distension.
Nausea	Queasiness or sick sensation; a feeling of the need to vomit.

Source: Modified from Talley NJ, Stanghellini V, Heading RC, et al.: Functional gastroduodenal disorders. *Gut* 1999;45:1137–1142.

are noninvasive tests used to diagnose neuromuscular disorders such as gastric dysrhythmias and gastroparesis in these patients. If the EGG or gastric emptying tests are abnormal, then the cause of the dyspepsia symptoms can be placed on an objective and pathophysiological basis and a rational approach to treatment can be designed.

Gastric Neuromuscular Dysfunction and Dyspepsia

Nausea, bloating, and abdominal discomfort are associated with a number of gastric neuromuscular abnormalities. These abnormalities include disorders of fundic relaxation, gastric dysrhythmias, antral hypomotility, pylorospasm, and disturbed fundic-corpus distribution of meals.[33,38] Noninvasive tests lend themselves to clinical studies and have high acceptability by patients. The noninvasive EGG and gastric emptying studies are complementary tests used to diagnose and categorize patients with the dyspepsia symptoms described.

The Electrogastrogram and Water Load Test

The EGG and water load test provide a provocative test of stomach distention and gastric myoelectrical activity.[31] An overview of the test protocol is shown in Figure 6.2. The patient or volunteer fasts after midnight. The patient eats one piece of unbuttered toast and drinks 4 oz. of apple juice. This light snack of approximately 200 Kcal prevents severe hunger (and sometimes nausea) and also abolishes phase III contractions that may occur during prolonged fasting. The standard snack also ensures a consistent baseline EGG. After the standard snack, the subject fasts for 2 hours until the EGG and water load test are performed.

A 15-minute baseline EGG is recorded, and then the water load test begins. From 1.0 to 1.5 L of cool (23°C) spring water is set aside for this test. The subject is asked to drink the water over a 5-minute period until he or she feels "full." The following instructions are used to explain the water load test to the patient: *"I now want you to drink the water from this cup until you feel full. You will have 5 minutes to drink water until you feel your stomach is full. I will tell you when 2 minutes and 4 minutes are up and when there are 30 seconds remaining in the 5-minute period. There is no correct amount to ingest and you may stop before the 5 minutes if your stomach feels full. Please begin now."* The subject should feel no pressure

EGG with Water Load Test

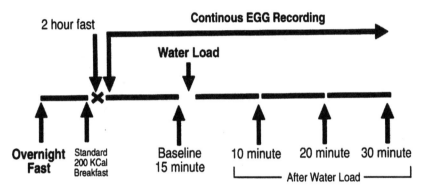

Figure 6.2. Outline of the water load test and electrogastrogram (EGG) recordings. After an overnight fast, a standard snack, and a 2-hour fast, the EGG with water load test is performed. After the water load test, the EGG is recorded for an additional 30 minutes, during which the gastric electrical response and symptoms are measured.

to finish the entire container of water but to drink only until he or she feels full. The volume of water consumed is recorded in ounces or milliliters. The EGG recording period continues for an additional 30 minutes after the ingestion of the water load is completed. Symptom scores and visceral sensations are measured at 10, 20, and 30 minutes after the water is ingested. Healthy volunteers consume approximately 600 ml of water during the water load test.[31] Healthy subjects feel full but report no nausea or bloating symptoms during the 30 minutes after ingestion of water.[31] Figures 3.13, 3.14, and 3.15 show examples of a normal EGG response to the water load test in healthy individuals. Caloric or solid test meals may also used during EGG recordings.[32,37]

The EGG test diagnoses gastric dysrhythmias (tachygastria, bradygastria, or mixed dysrhythmia) or the presence of normal gastric myoelectrical activity.[39] Gastric dysrhythmias are recorded in a number of clinical conditions where nausea and vomiting are prominent symptoms. The presence of gastric dysrhythmias represents an objective pathophysiological finding that may mediate upper GI symptoms and represents a target for treatments.[39] Examples of these dysrhythmias are shown in Figures 6.3, 6.4, and 6.5. Another abnormal EGG pattern is the loss of baseline 3-cpm EGG signals after the water load or caloric test meals. The EGG signal "flatlines" after the test meal and 3-cpm signal is lost, but neither tachygastrias nor bradygastrias are elicited. An example of this pattern is shown in Figure 6.6.

The EGG test can be further analyzed by determining whether the patient was able to ingest a normal volume of water. The volume of water ingested by healthy volunteers in 5 minutes averaged 557 ml, whereas patients with functional dyspepsia ingested only 357 ml and felt full.[31] The volume of water ingested during the water load test provides an indirect assessment of the ability of the stomach to accommodate or relax until fullness is experienced; that is, the stomach must relax during the 5-minute period to receive and accommodate the ingested volume. Stomach relaxation in response to the water load test includes relaxation of the antrum, corpus, and fundus. The water load test is distinct from barostat testing during which only fundic contraction and relaxation are assessed. A patient with a gastric dysrhythmia (or a normal EGG pattern) may have a normal or abnormal water load test (Fig. 6.7).

Figure 6.7 illustrates the results of the EGG and water load test in patients with unexplained upper GI symptoms. First, if the patient has a gastric dysrhythmia (with or without an abnormal water load test),

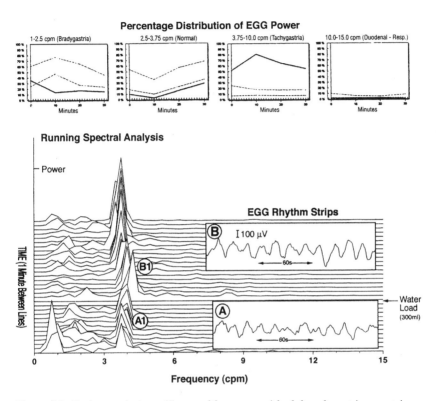

Percentage Distribution of EGG Power

1-2.5 cpm (Bradygastria)   2.5-3.75 cpm (Normal)   3.75-10.0 cpm (Tachygastria)   10.0-15.0 cpm (Duodenal - Resp.)

Minutes   Minutes   Minutes   Minutes

Running Spectral Analysis

Power

EGG Rhythm Strips

B   I 100 µV

B1

60s

A1   A

60s

Water Load (300ml)

TIME (1 Minute Between Lines)

Frequency (cpm)

0   3   6   9   12   15

Figure 6.3. Tachygastria in a 45-year-old woman with delayed gastric emptying. Electrogastrogram (EGG) rhythm strips, running spectral analysis (RSA), and percentage distribution of EGG power graphs are shown. The EGG rhythm strip (A) from baseline shows a 4-cpm rhythm. The patient ingested 300 ml of water as part of the water load test, and the EGG rhythm strip (B) shows persistence of the 4-cpm EGG rhythm, a clear tachygastria. The RSA shows peaks at baseline (A1) near 4 cpm. After the water load test, the 4-cpm activity increases briefly and is followed by a trend toward 3.5-cpm peaks during the remainder of the recording. The percentage distribution of EGG power shows increased tachygastria at baseline and throughout the water load test. The percentage of power in the bradygastria range is below normal, and the normal 3-cpm activity is below normal throughout the test.

109

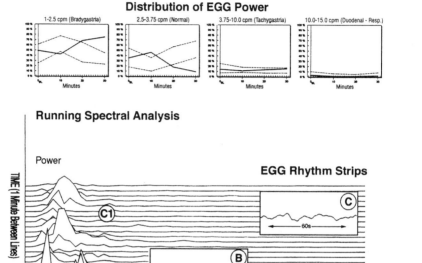

Figure 6.4. Bradygastria with normal water load. Electrogastrogram (EGG) rhythm strips, running spectral analysis (RSA), and percentage distribution of EGG power from a patient with unexplained nausea. The baseline EGG rhythm strip shows normal 3-cpm activity (A) and 3-cpm peaks are also shown in the RSA at baseline (A1). After ingestion of 530 ml water, there is a 2- to 2.5-cpm EGG response in the first 10 minutes (B) and peaks in the RSA are seen in the 2.5- to 3-cpm range (B1). However, thereafter, there is very little 3-cpm activity in the EGG (C). Most of the peaks in the RSA are in the 1- to 2-cpm bradygastria range (C1). The percent distribution of EGG power graphs mirror these changes with an initial increase in 3-cpm activity 10 minutes after ingestion of water, but progressively less 3-cpm activity thereafter. On the other hand, there were no increases in the percentage distribution of tachygastria or duodenal activity, but the bradygastria activity increased abnormally 20 and 30 minutes after the ingestion of water.

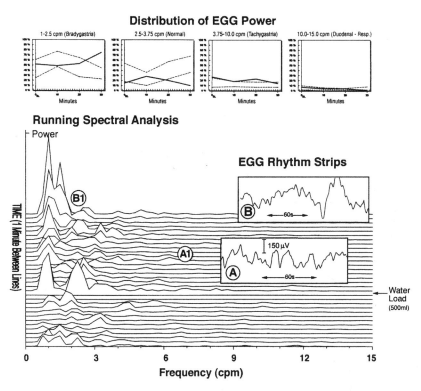

Figure 6.5. Mixed dysrhythmia with normal water load test. Electrogastrogram (EGG) rhythm strips, running spectral analysis (RSA), and percentage distribution of EGG power graphs in a patient with gastroesophageal reflux symptoms and bloating and nausea. The EGG rhythm strip after ingestion of water at (*A*) shows a 6- to 7-cpm tachygastria. Very small peaks are seen at 6 to 7 cpm in the RSA (A1). By the end of the recording, there are large waves at 1 to 2 cpm in the EGG signal (*B*) and also in the RSA (B1). The percentage distribution of EGG power graphs also show increased 3-cpm activity at 10 minutes after the ingestion of water, but then the 3-cpm activity decreased below normal. The percentage tachygastria at 20-minute and bradygastria activity at 30-minute ingestion of water are increased.

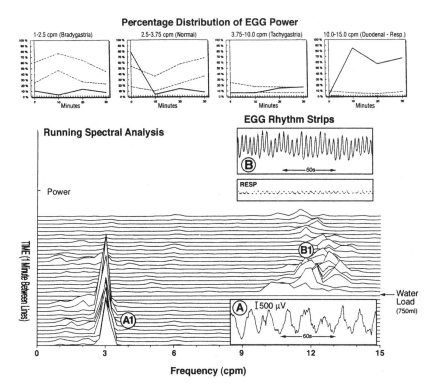

Figure 6.6. Loss of 3-cpm activity after water load test. Electrogastrogram (EGG) rhythm strips, running spectral analysis (RSA), and percentage distribution of EGG power are shown in a patient with postprandial bloating and nausea. The EGG rhythm strip (A) recorded from baseline shows a clear 3-cpm EGG signal. After ingestion of water, the EGG rhythm strip (B) shows no 3-cpm rhythm, but only a 12 per minute respiratory rhythm. Respiration (Resp) is shown below the EGG rhythm strip. The respiration rate is 12/min. The RSA shows clear peaks at baseline at 3 cpm (A1), but after ingestion of a normal water load (750 ml), the 3-cpm peaks disappear. The peaks in the RSA (B1) are at 12 to 13 cpm, the rate of respiration. The percent distribution of EGG power in the 3-cpm range is 80% during baseline. However, after ingestion of the water, 3-cpm activity decreases to below the normal range. At the same time, there is marked increase in the percentage of EGG power in the respiration range. There is no increased percentage activity in the tachygastria or bradygastria ranges.

112

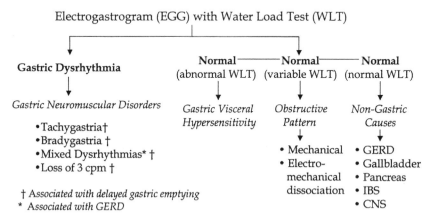

Electrogastrogram (EGG) with Water Load Test (WLT)

Gastric Dysrhythmia

Gastric Neuromuscular Disorders

- Tachygastria†
- Bradygastria †
- Mixed Dysrhythmias* †
- Loss of 3 cpm †

† *Associated with delayed gastric emptying*
* *Associated with GERD*

Normal—————Normal—————Normal
(abnormal WLT) (variable WLT) (normal WLT)

*Gastric Visceral
Hypersensitivity*

*Obstructive
Pattern*

- Mechanical
- Electro-
  mechanical
  dissociation

*Non-Gastric
Causes*

- GERD
- Gallbladder
- Pancreas
- IBS
- CNS

Figure 6.7. Results of electrogastrogram (EGG) with water load test (WLT). In patients with functional dyspepsia symptoms, a diagnosis of gastric dysrhythmia indicates a gastric neuromuscular disorder that can be characterized as tachygastria, bradygastria, or mixed dysrhythmias or loss of 3-cpm activity after a test meal. A normal EGG with an abnormal WLT suggests gastric visceral hypersensitivity, a disorder that may include the abnormalities of gastric stretch or visceral hypersensitivity. A normal 3-cpm EGG with variable WLT results may reflect obstruction of the gastrointestinal tract. In these cases, the 3-cpm activity usually exhibits very clear, high-amplitude 3-cpm waves. If 3-cpm amplitudes are normal but gastroparesis is present, then electromechanical dissociation is diagnosed. Finally, if the patient has a normal EGG rhythm and a normal WLT, the stomach may not be the source of symptoms. Nongastric causes of symptoms should be considered and these include atypical GERD, gallbladder disease, pancreatic disease, irritable bowel syndrome, and central nervous system disorders.

then a myoelectrical abnormality is established. Figures 6.3, 6.4, 6.5, and 6.6 are examples of tachygastria, bradygastria, mixed dysrhythmias, and loss of 3-cpm activity, respectively. The poor water load volume also indicates dysfunction in the stretch or relaxation of the muscular wall of the stomach. The diagnosis of a specific gastric dysrhythmia is also useful because patients with tachygastria have poorer gastric emptying compared with patients with bradygastria or normal 3-cpm EGG patterns (Fig. 6.8).

Second, if the patient has a 3-cpm EGG rhythm (Fig. 6.7), then there are several diagnostic possibilities to consider. Figures 6.9, 6.10, and 6.11 show examples of different types of 3-cpm EGG patterns. If a normal EGG response and a normal water load test volume are found (Fig. 6.9), then gastric myoelectrical rhythm and the ability of the stomach to relax to receive the volume of water are normal. These patients are unlikely to have a delay in gastric emptying. Their symptoms may be due to a nongastric cause. Nongastric causes of symptoms include atypical gastroesophageal reflux disease (GERD), gallbladder or pancreatic disease, irritable bowel syndrome, or central nervous system disorders. For example, patients with unexplained chronic nausea due to occult GERD had normal 3-cpm EGG patterns and normal gastric emptying; these patients had abnormal 24-hour esophageal pH studies and nausea correlated with acid reflux events.[40] Thus, a 24-hour esophageal pH study, gallbladder emptying study, or computed tomography scan of the head may be indicated in certain patients.

If the EGG rhythm is the normal 3-cpm pattern but the water load test is abnormal (less than 300 ml consumed), then gastric myoelectrical activity is normal and gastric relaxation or stretch is abnormal. This group of patients may have a form of gastric visceral hypersensitivity. However, the abnormal water load test also suggests that abnormalities of relaxation of the neuromuscular wall of the stomach may be present. These patients may benefit from muscle relaxants such as dicyclomine, calcium channel blockers, or nitrates.

Finally, if a 3-cpm EGG rhythm is present but gastric emptying is delayed, then either electrical-mechanical dissociation (Fig. 6.10) or mechanical obstruction (Fig. 6.11) of the stomach is present. This category is uncommon (<4% of patients with functional dyspepsia). Results of a solid-phase gastric emptying are needed to confirm gastroparesis.[31] Electromechanical dissociation is defined by an abnormal solid-phase, gastric emptying study and a normal 3-cpm EGG. Prokinetic agents such as bethanechol or erythromycin may be helpful in these cases

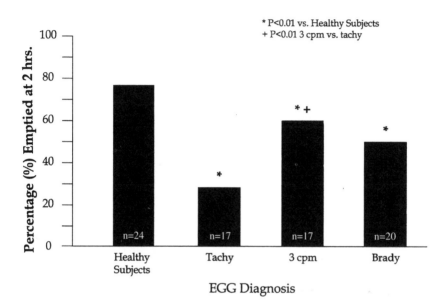

Figure 6.8. Solid-phase gastric emptying and electrogastrogram (EGG) test results in patients with chronic nausea and vomiting. The average percentage of
scrambled eggs emptied at 2 hours is approximately 75% in healthy subjects.
Gastric emptying results in patients with tachygastrias (Tachy), bradygastrias
(Brady), and 3-cpm EGG diagnoses are shown. Patients with tachygastria had significantly reduced gastric emptying compared with the healthy subjects and with
the patients with normal 3-cpm EGG results.

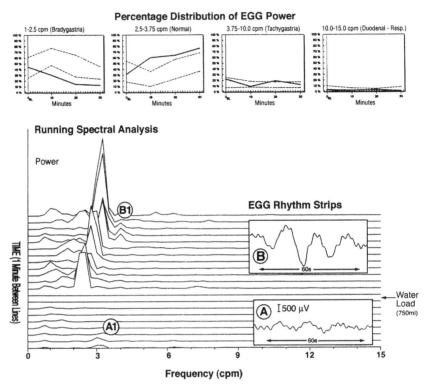

Figure 6.9. Normal electrogastrogram (EGG) and water load test recorded from a 16-year-old high school sophomore with persistent nausea and vomiting. EGG rhythm strips, running spectral analysis (RSA), and percentage distribution of EGG power are shown. The EGG rhythm strip at (A) shows a 3-cpm EGG signal. After ingestion of the water load, clear 3-cpm EGG waves are seen (B). The RSA shows several tiny peaks at 3 cpm during baseline (A1). After the water load test, there is the temporary frequency dip to approximately 2.5 cpm and then a steady increase in the peaks at 3 cpm (B1). The percentage distribution of EGG power shows normal percentages at baseline. After ingestion of water, there is an increase in 3-cpm activity above the normal range during the minutes after the water load test. There are no increased tachygastria or bradygastria percentages. Thus, this is a normal EGG and water load test. A CT scan of the abdomen showed uretero-pelvic obstruction and cystic dilation of the nonfunctioning left kidney. Nausea and vomiting resolved after nephrectomy.

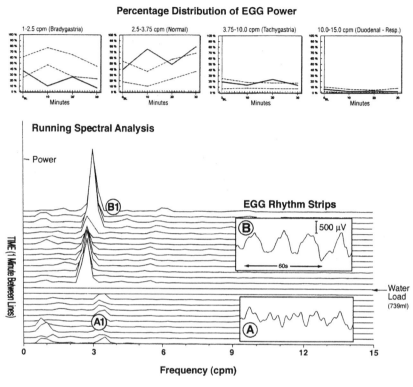

Figure 6.10. Normal electrogastrogram (EGG) pattern recorded from a 55-year-old patient with diabetes mellitus, marked bloating symptoms, and gastroparesis. This is an example of electromechanical dissociation. The EGG rhythm strips, running spectral analysis (RSA), and percentage distribution of EGG power are shown. The baseline EGG rhythm strip (A) shows 3-cpm waves are present. After ingestion of 750 ml of water, the EGG rhythm strip (B) shows clear 3-cpm EGG waves. The RSA at baseline shows a series of peaks at approximately 3.5 cpm (A1). After ingestion of water, there is a slight frequency dip and then persistent peaks at approximately 3 cpm (B1). The percentage distribution of EGG power graphs show normal percentages at baseline. After ingestion of water, there is an increase in the percentage of EGG power in the 3-cpm range at 10 and 30 minutes after ingestion of water. There is a slight increase in tachygastria percentage at 20 minutes, but this reflects the harmonics at 5 and 6 cpm, which are also seen in the RSA.

117

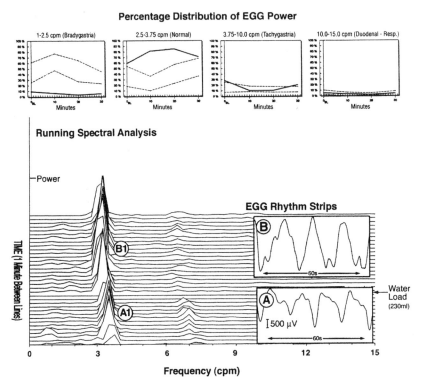

Percentage Distribution of EGG Power

| 1-2.5 cpm (Bradygastria) | 2.5-3.75 cpm (Normal) | 3.75-10.0 cpm (Tachygastria) | 10.0-15.0 cpm (Duodenal - Resp.) |

Figure 6.11. Normal electrogastrogram (EGG) pattern recorded in a 45-year-old woman with pyloric stenosis and gastroparesis. EGG rhythm strips, running spectral analysis (RSA), and percentage distribution of EGG power are shown. The baseline EGG rhythm strip shows clear 3-cpm high-amplitude waves. The patient was able to ingest only a small amount of water, and the EGG recorded after water ingestion continues to show high-amplitude 3-cpm signals. The RSA shows clear peaks during baseline at approximately 3.5 cpm (A1), and after the ingestion of water, there is a rigid persistence of these frequency peaks (B1). The percentage distribution of EGG power shows that there is increased 3-cpm activity at baseline and that this is sustained throughout the post water load portion of the study. There is no frequency dip. The percentages in the bradygastria or tachygastria ranges are normal.

because they stimulate smooth muscle contractions presumably at the normal 3-cpm rhythm. In mechanical obstruction, however, the EGG waves are distinct with very high amplitudes and extremely consistent 3-cpm EGG signals (Fig. 6.11). If the EGG shows this obstruction pattern, then further testing is indicated with endoscopy or barium studies to identify the site of obstruction.[11]

Thus, the EGG and water load test provide useful clinical information about the myoelectrical activity and capacity (relaxation) of the stomach. The EGG recording with water load test is analogous to the ECG recording with exercise treadmill test. The baseline may or may not be abnormal, but the response of the stomach to the provocative stimulation of water loading is the measure of interest. The EGG categories described earlier also help to direct therapeutic approaches or further diagnostic tests as shown in Figure 6.12.

Electrogastrographic and Gastric Emptying Tests. Patients with gastric dysrhythmias and upper GI symptoms may or may not have delayed gastric emptying. Similarly, patients with atrial fibrillation with palpitations and chest discomfort may or may not have impaired cardiac output. Patients with bradygastria have normal or near-normal gastric emptying rates, whereas patients with tachygastrias have poorer gastric emptying (Fig. 6.8). Patients with dyspepsia symptoms can be further categorized on a pathophysiological basis by combining the EGG and gastric emptying test results. An objective and pathophysiological basis for dyspepsia symptoms contributes to understanding the patient's symptoms and to designing rational therapeutic approaches.

Figure 6.13 shows the results of EGG and gastric emptying studies in 24 patients with unexplained dysmotility-like dyspepsia. Approximately 60% of these patients had gastric dysrhythmias and 40% had normal gastric myoelectrical rhythms in response to the water load. Gastric emptying was delayed in 17% (*category 1*) but was normal in more than 80% of these symptomatic patients. Category 1 patients with gastric dysrhythmia and gastroparesis have severe electrical and contractile abnormalities of the stomach. These patients frequently require various prokinetic drugs and extensive dietary consultation and may require other nutritional support with enteral feeding or total parenteral nutrition.

On the other hand, 42% of these patients with dyspepsia had a gastric dysrhythmia only (*category 2*). Gastric emptying studies in these patients were normal. Thus, the patients in category 2 have a lesser

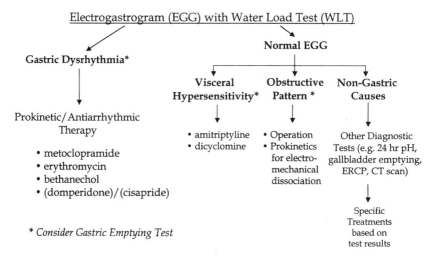

Electrogastrogram (EGG) with Water Load Test (WLT)

Normal EGG

Gastric Dysrhythmia*

Prokinetic/Antiarrhythmic
Therapy

- metoclopramide
- erythromycin
- bethanechol
- (domperidone)/(cisapride)

* Consider Gastric Emptying Test

**Visceral
Hypersensitivity***

- amitriptyline
- dicyclomine

**Obstructive
Pattern ***

- Operation
- Prokinetics
  for electro-
  mechanical
  dissociation

**Non-Gastric
Causes**

Other Diagnostic
Tests (e.g. 24 hr pH,
gallbladder emptying,
ERCP, CT scan)

Specific
Treatments
based on
test results

Figure 6.12. An approach to treatment of patients with investigated dyspepsia symptoms based on electrogastrogram and water load test results. Patients with gastric dysrhythmia may be treated with prokinetic drugs that also have antiarrhythmic characteristics. In contrast, patients with a normal EGG may have visceral hypersensitivity and trials of amitriptyline or dicyclomine may be used. If an obstructive EGG pattern is determined and a specific obstructing lesion is found, then a surgical operation is indicated. Prokinetics are used to treat electrical mechanical dissociation. If nongastric causes of symptoms are considered a possibility, then other diagnostic tests may be indicated and specific treatments are based on the test results.

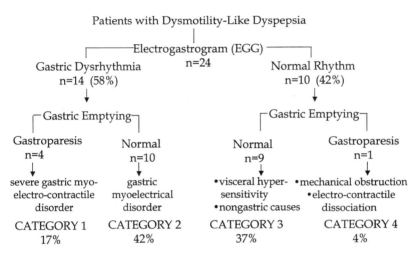

Patients with Dysmotility-Like Dyspepsia

Electrogastrogram (EGG)
n=24

Gastric Dysrhythmia
n=14 (58%)

Normal Rhythm
n=10 (42%)

Gastric Emptying

Gastric Emptying

Gastroparesis
n=4

Normal
n=10

Normal
n=9

Gastroparesis
n=1

severe gastric myo-
electro-contractile
disorder

gastric
myoelectrical
disorder

• visceral hyper-
sensitivity
• nongastric causes

• mechanical obstruction
• electro-contractile
dissociation

CATEGORY 1
17%

CATEGORY 2
42%

CATEGORY 3
37%

CATEGORY 4
4%

Figure 6.13. Electrogastrogram (EGG) and gastric emptying test results in 24 patients with dysmotility-like dyspepsia; 58% of these patients had gastric dysrhythmias and 42% had normal EGGs. Category 1 patients have severe gastric myoelectrical and contractile disorders, whereas category 2 patients have gastric myoelectrical disorders only. Seventeen percent of the patients were in category 1, and 42% were in category 2. On the other hand, 37% of the patients had normal EGGs and normal gastric emptying, indicating either visceral hypersensitivity or non-gastric causes of these symptoms. Only 4% of the patients had a normal rhythm and delayed gastric emptying (category 4).

degree of neuromuscular injury compared with category 1 patients. Treatment approaches to these patients are similar to but usually less intensive than treatment for category 1 patients.

Thirty-seven percent of the patients with functional dyspepsia had a normal EGG test *and* a normal gastric emptying studies (category 3). These patients have either gastric visceral hypersensitivity or nongastric causes of their symptoms. Treatment for visceral hypersensitivity with amitriptyline or further diagnostic tests are rational approaches for the management of these patients.

Finally, *category 4* patients with normal EGG rhythms and delayed gastric emptying are uncommon. This group requires medical treatment if electromechanical dissociation is present or further diagnostic tests to exclude obstructions, as described earlier.

The results of EGG tests and gastric emptying tests provide insights into the various gastric neuromuscular abnormalities present in patients with common unexplained upper GI symptoms. The EGG and gastric emptying tests were used in evaluating gastric neuromuscular dysfunction in two other common groups of patients: (1) patients with GERD *and* functional dyspepsia symptoms (GERD+) and (2) patients with unexplained nausea and vomiting.

Fifty-four patients with unexplained nausea and vomiting underwent an EGG with water load test and gastric emptying test. Figure 6.14 shows the percentage of patients in the four categories: 37% had severe electrocontractile abnormalities (category 1), 30% had gastric dysrhythmias only (category 2), 22% had normal EGGs and normal emptying (category 3), and 10% had normal EGGs and gastroparesis (category 4).[41] Compared with the functional dyspepsia patients described earlier (Fig. 6.13), more patients presenting with unexplained nausea and vomiting had severe gastric neuromuscular dysfunction (categories 1 and 2). The EGG diagnoses in these patients with unexplained nausea and vomiting were normal in 32%, tachygastria in 30%, and bradygastria in 38% of the patients. Figure 6.8 shows the EGG diagnosis and the percentage of the solid phase test meal emptied in 2 hours. Patients with tachygastria had significantly poorer gastric emptying compared with patients with 3-cpm or bradygastria EGG patterns. Considerable variability in emptying occurred, however, reflecting the fact that some symptomatic patients with dysrhythmias have normal gastric emptying rates.

Electrogastrographic recordings with the water load test and solid-phase gastric emptying tests were performed in 67 patients with GERD+. The results are summarized in Figure 6.15. These studies indicated that

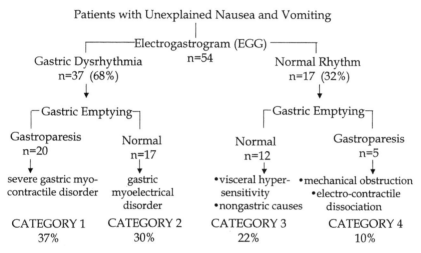

Patients with Unexplained Nausea and Vomiting
|
┌────────Electrogastrogram (EGG)────────┐
Gastric Dysrhythmia   n=54   Normal Rhythm
n=37 (68%)   n=17 (32%)
↓   ↓

┌─Gastric Emptying─┐   ┌─Gastric Emptying─┐

Gastroparesis   Normal   Normal   Gastroparesis
n=20   n=17   n=12   n=5
↓   ↓   ↓   ↓
severe gastric myo-   gastric   •visceral hyper- •mechanical obstruction
contractile disorder myoelectrical   sensitivity   •electro-contractile
                      disorder   •nongastric causes dissociation

CATEGORY 1   CATEGORY 2   CATEGORY 3   CATEGORY 4
37%   30%   22%   10%

Figure 6.14. Electrogastrogram (EGG) and gastric emptying results in 54 patients with unexplained nausea and vomiting. In this group of patients, 68% had gastric dysrhythmias and 32% had normal EGG rhythms. Thirty-seven percent of these patients had delayed gastric emptying (category 1), and 30% of the patients with gastric dysrhythmias had normal emptying (category 2). In this patient population, 22% had normal EGG and normal gastric emptying (category 3), whereas 10% had normal rhythm and delayed gastric emptying (category 4). Four of these five patients in category 4 were eventually found to have specific sites of obstruction of the stomach or duodenum.

123

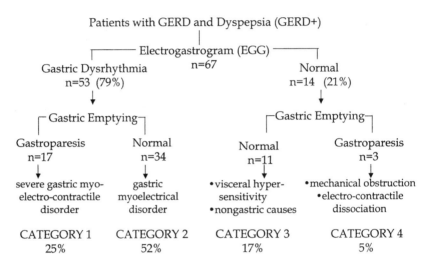

Patients with GERD and Dyspepsia (GERD+)

┌────────── Electrogastrogram (EGG) ──────────┐
                        n=67
Gastric Dysrhythmia   Normal
n=53 (79%)   n=14 (21%)

┌─Gastric Emptying─┐   ┌─Gastric Emptying─┐

Gastroparesis   Normal   Normal   Gastroparesis
n=17   n=34   n=11   n=3

severe gastric myo- gastric   • visceral hyper- • mechanical obstruction
electro-contractile myoelectrical   sensitivity   • electro-contractile
disorder   disorder   • nongastric causes dissociation

CATEGORY 1   CATEGORY 2   CATEGORY 3   CATEGORY 4
25%   52%   17%   5%

Figure 6.15. Electrogastrogram (EGG) and gastric emptying results in 67 patients with gastroesophageal reflux disease and dyspepsia symptoms (GERD+); 79% of these patients had a gastric dysrhythmias, and 21% had normal EGGs. Twenty-five percent of the patients had severe gastric electrical and contractile disorders (category 1), whereas 52% had gastric dysrhythmias only (category 2). A small percentage of patients had category 3 or category 4 pathophysiology.

almost 80% of the patients with GERD+ had gastric dysrhythmias.[42] Mixed dysrhythmias were common in patients with GERD+. Twenty-five percent of these patients were category 1 on the basis of their EGG and gastric emptying test results. Thus, the patients with GERD+ had more severe gastric neuromuscular dysfunction compared with patients with dysmotility-like dyspepsia symptoms alone, but as a group they had less severe dysfunction compared with the patients with chronic unexplained nausea and vomiting. Fifty-two percent of the patients with GERD+ had a gastric dysrhythmia only (category 2). On the other hand, only 30% of the patients with unexplained nausea and vomiting were in category 2, but 42% of the patients with dysmotility-like dyspepsia had a dysrhythmia only. In regard to the distribution of normal 3-cpm activity, only 17% of the patients with GERD+ were in category 3. In contrast, 37% of the dysmotility-like dyspepsia group and 22% of the unexplained nausea and vomiting patients were in category 3. Finally, only 5% of the patients with GERD+ were in category 4. Thus, patients with different presenting symptoms had different distributions of gastric neuromuscular dysfunction.

To summarize, the EGG with water load test diagnoses gastric dysrhythmias (tachygastria, bradygastria, mixed dysrhythmia, poor 3-cpm response to meal) or normal gastric myoelectrical activity. Furthermore, an indirect assessment of gastric capacity (i.e., relaxation) is determined by the volume of water ingested during the water load test. On the basis of the EGG results, different treatment approaches or further diagnostic tests can be determined. The gastric emptying study provides evidence for severe gastric neuromuscular dysfunction and complements the EGG test results. For some patients, further testing with barostat balloons to determine fundic compliance or catheter studies to determine antroduodenal motility may be indicated.

Treatment of Gastric Neuromuscular Disorders Based on Pathophysiological Categories

Therapeutic options for the treatment of gastric neuromuscular disorders are increasing but remain limited.[35] Category 1 and 2 patients with gastric dysrhythmias (with or without gastroparesis) are treated with drugs designed to increase contractility of the corpus and antrum and promote gastric emptying ("prokinetic" agents) (Fig. 6.16). Presently available prokinetic agents also can improve gastric dysrhythmias, as

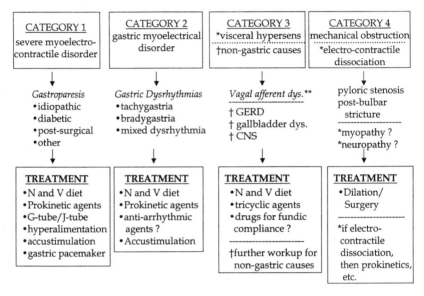

Figure 6.16. Summary of the approach to patients with unexplained nausea and dyspepsia symptoms based on electrogastrogram and gastric emptying results, pathophysiology, and treatments. N and V, nausea and vomiting; G-tube, gastrostomy; J-tube, jejunostomy tube; hypersens, hypersensitivity; GERD, gastroesophageal reflux disease; CNS, central nervous system.

shown later, and are antiarrhythmic agents in some patients. Prokinetic drugs and agents that affect neurosensory activity are listed in Table 6.3. Because the precise neuromuscular cause(s) of the underlying gastric dysrhythmias (or delayed emptying) is not known, drug selection is an empiric process at this time. Several drugs may be tried before a drug that reduces symptoms is found. Each drug should be given a trial for 3 to 4 weeks' duration.

Category 1 and 2 patients with gastric dysrhythmias may respond to these prokinetic agents that also have antiarrhythmic properties. Figure 6.17 shows correction of tachygastria and establishment of normal 3-cpm rhythm after metoclopramide therapy, a drug with actions on dopamine$_2$ receptors and 5-hydroxytryptamine$_3$ (5-HT$_3$) and 5-HT$_4$ receptors. Figure 6.18 shows the effect of domperidone on bradygastria recorded from a patient with diabetic gastroparesis. Over time, the bradygastria is converted to a 3-cpm EGG rhythm during domperidone treatment. Figure 6.19 shows the effects of bethanecol, a muscarinic receptor agonist, in improving 3-cpm EGG activity. Figure 6.20 shows a bradygastria in a patient with idiopathic gastroparesis. The patient was given the 5-HT$_4$ agonist cisapride (10 mg four times daily), and over a 6-week treatment period the bradygastria was eradicated and normal 3-cpm EGG signals developed. The patient's symptoms were markedly improved. Figure 6.21 shows improvement in normal 3-cpm gastric myoelectrical activity in a patient with probable tachygastria who received tegaserod (a partial 5-HT$_4$ agonist), 6 mg two times daily for 3 months.

Another example of improvement in gastric dysrhythmias and improvements in symptoms is shown in Figure 6.22. Before operation, the patient had a bradygastria as shown in the EGG inset in this figure. The running spectral analysis (RSA) also shows many peaks in the bradygastria range. In this patient, gastric dysrhythmias were reversed after correction of chronic mesenteric artery ischemia. After bypass grafting of the superior mesenteric artery and the celiac artery was performed, a normal 3-cpm EGG pattern was reestablished. The postoperative EGG shows regular 3-cpm EGG waves and increased 3-cpm peaks in the RSA. The patient's upper GI symptoms and delayed gastric emptying resolved after revascularization.

Figure 6.23 shows the RSA from an EGG recorded before and after radiofrequency ablation (RFA) with the STRETTA procedure in a patient with GERD and dyspepsia symptoms (GERD+). The pre-STRETTA EGG shows a tachygastria pattern in the EGG rhythm strip

Table 6.3. Drugs Used to Treat Symptoms Associated with Gastroparesis and Gastric Neuromuscular Disorders

Drug	Mechanisms of Action	Dosage	Side Effects
Prokinetic Agents			
Metoclopramide	Dopamine (D_2) receptor antagonist, 5-HT_3 receptor antagonist, 5-HT_4 agonist	5–10 mg before meals and at bedtime	Extrapyramidal symptoms, dystonic reactions, anxiety, drowsiness, hyperprolactinemia
Cisapride	5-HT_4 receptor agonist	5–10 mg before meals	Cardiac dysrhythmias, diarrhea, abdominal discomfort
Erythromycin	Motilin agonist	125–250 mg four times daily	Nausea, diarrhea, abdominal cramps, rash
Domperidone	D_2-receptor antagonist (peripheral)	10–20 mg before meals and at bedtime	Hyperprolactinemia
Tegaserod*	Partial 5-HT_4 agonist	6 mg two times daily or 2 mg three times daily	Diarrhea, abdominal pain
*Neurosensory Agents**			
Droperidol	Central dopamine antagonist	2.5–5.0 mg IV	Sedation, hypotension
Alprazolam	Central nervous system sites, benzodiazepine	0.5 mg PO	Drowsiness, lightheadedness
Clonidine	Central α-adrenergic agonist	0.1–0.3 mg PO	Dry mouth, drowsiness, dizziness
Alosetron	5-HT_3 antagonist	1.0 mg PO	Constipation, ischemic colitis

*Drugs are used empirically as few or no controlled trials are available.

A

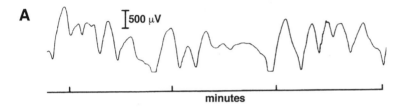

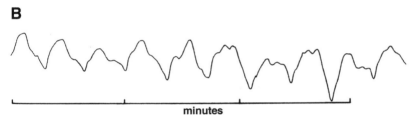

Figure 6.17. Effect of metoclopramide on tachygastria recorded from a patient with idiopathic gastroparesis. (*A*) Tachygastria before treatment. (*B*) Eradication of the dysrhythmia and establishment of 3-cpm waves 20 minutes after the patient was given 20 mg of metoclopramide by mouth.

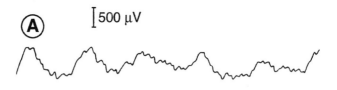

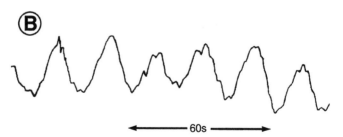

Figure 6.18. Effect of domperidone (10 mg, PO) on electrogastrogram (EGG) signals in a patient with unexplained nausea and vomiting. The baseline EGG shows unstable rhythm (*A*). Twenty-five minutes after the domperidone was ingested, a clear 3-cpm EGG rhythm developed (*B*).

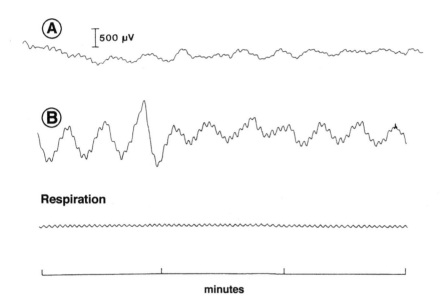

Figure 6.19. Effect of bethanecol on electrogastrogram (EGG) activity in a patient with chronic nausea. (*A*) Fasting EGG pattern with some 3-cpm activity. (*B*) Clear 3-cpm EGG rhythm recorded 30 minutes after the patient ingested 10 mg of bethanecol by mouth.

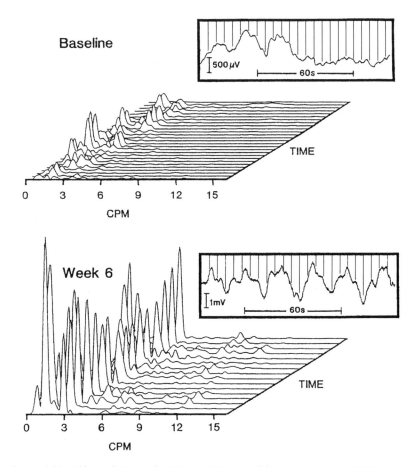

Figure 6.20. Effect of cisapride (10 mg QID) on electrogastrogram (EGG) activity in a patient with chronic nausea and vomiting. The baseline EGG shows 1- to 2-cpm waves. The running spectral analysis (RSA) at baseline shows some peaks at 3 cpm but larger peaks at 1 to 2 cpm. EGG rhythm strip from week 6 of cisapride treatment shows steady improvement in the 3-cpm rhythm. Similarly, there are increased peaks at 3 cpm in the RSA. The patient's symptoms of nausea and vomiting improved during cisapride treatment.

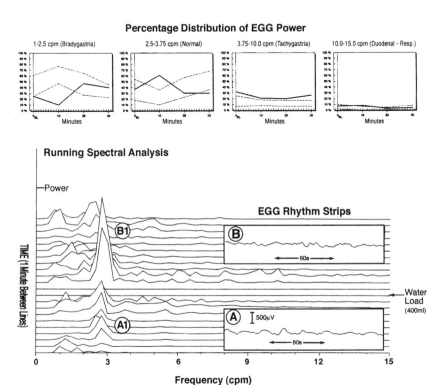

Figure 6.21.A Effect of tegaserod (6 mg BID PO) on EGG activity in a woman with recurrent nausea, early satiety, and mildly delayed gastric emptying. EGG rhythm strips, running spectral analysis (RSA), and percentage distribution of EGG power during baseline are shown *before* treatment. The EGG rhythm strips (A and B) show a variety of dysrhythmias. The RSA shows some peaks at 3 cpm at baseline (A1), but a poor response to the water load with loss of 3-cpm peaks and increased tachygastria throughout the test is seen (B1). The percent distribution of EGG power shows some 3-cpm activity, but mild tachygastria is present throughout the test.

133

Percentage Distribution of EGG Power

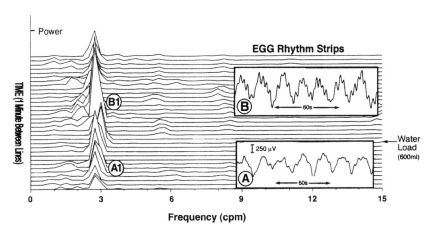

Running Spectral Analysis

Figure 6.21B. EGG rhythm strips, RSA, and percentage distribution of EGG power from the same patient 3 months after receiving tegaserod 6 mg BID. The EGG rhythm strips now show clear 3-cpm EGG signals before (A) and after (B) the water load test. Increased water was ingested during this EGG test compared with before treatment. Furthermore, the RSA shows very regular peaks at 3 cpm before (A1) and after (B1) the water load test. The percentage distribution of EGG power shows increased 3 cpm activity 10, 20, and 30 minutes after ingestion of the water and tachygastria activity is within the normal range. The patient had improvement in the dyspepsia symptoms during treatment.

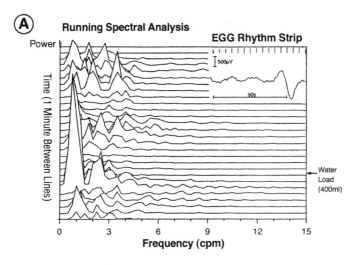

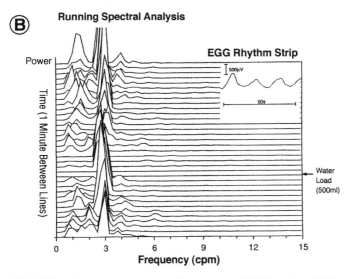

Figure 6.22. Effect of mesenteric revascularization on EGG activity. (*A*) Preoperative electrogastrogram (EGG) (inset) and the running spectral analysis (RSA) of the EGG rhythm strip before and after a water load test. The EGG shows a 2-cpm bradygastria. The RSA shows very few peaks at 3 cpm. There are a predominance of peaks in the 1- to 2-cpm range. (*B*) Postoperative EGG (inset) and the RSA from the same patient. The EGG recording was obtained 6 months after revascularization. A 3-cpm normal rhythm is seen in the EGG, and many peaks at the normal 3 cpm range are seen in the RSA. Dyspepsia symptoms, nausea, and vomiting and gastroparesis resolved.

135

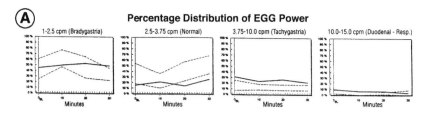

Percentage Distribution of EGG Power

1-2.5 cpm (Bradygastria)　　2.5-3.75 cpm (Normal)　　3.75-10.0 cpm (Tachygastria)　　10.0-15.0 cpm (Duodenal - Resp.)

Minutes　　Minutes　　Minutes　　Minutes

Running Spectral Analysis

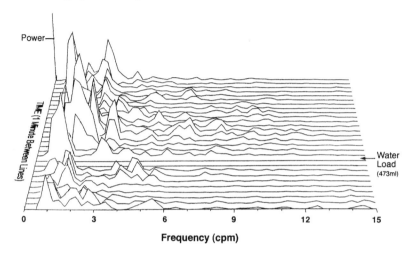

Power

TIME (1 Minute Between Lines)

Water Load (473ml)

0　　3　　6　　9　　12　　15

Frequency (cpm)

(B)

Percentage Distribution of EGG Power

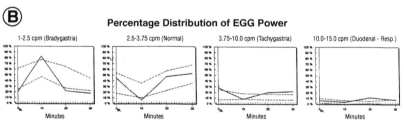

1-2.5 cpm (Bradygastria)　　2.5-3.75 cpm (Normal)　　3.75-10.0 cpm (Tachygastria)　　10.0-15.0 cpm (Duodenal - Resp.)

Minutes　　Minutes　　Minutes　　Minutes

Running Spectral Analysis

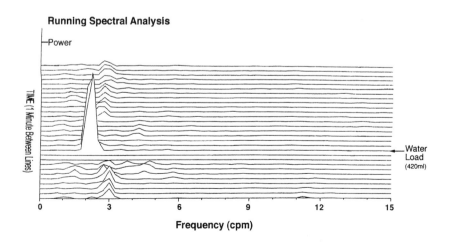

Power

TIME (1 Minute Between Lines)

Water Load (420ml)

0　　3　　6　　9　　12　　15

Frequency (cpm)

and multiple peaks in the tachygastria range in the RSA. The STRETTA procedure produces thermal injury to tissue in the lower esophageal sphincter region and cardia of the stomach. The EGG and RSA performed in this patient 6 months after the STRETTA procedure shows a normal 3-cpm EGG pattern, and the RSA is concordant with many peaks in the 3-cpm range. The beneficial effect of RFA on gastric dysrhythmias was found in approximately 30% of the patients with GERD+. The mechanism of this effect on gastric myoelectrical rhythm remains to be determined.

An example of an EGG recording in a patient with pyloric obstruction due to chronic peptic ulcer disease is shown in Figure 6.24. The regular 3-cpm EGG signal is clear. The RSA shows unvarying and extremely regular 3-cpm peaks. After the patient underwent vagotomy and antrectomy, the EGG signal decreased in amplitude and was more irregular. These changes are due to the effects of vagotomy and the antrectomy.[43] In addition, the remaining corpus with pacemaker activity is also affected by the vagotomy.[43]

Figure 6.23. Effect of radiofrequency ablation of the lower esophageal sphincter-cardia region in a patient with gastroesophageal reflux disease (GERD) and functional dyspepsia (GERDI+). (*A*) Running spectral analysis (RSA) of an EGG with water load test and percentage distribution of EGG power are shown. The RSA shows very little 3-cpm peaks at baseline. The subject ingested 473 ml of water as part of the water load test. A few peaks at 3 cpm are seen initially after the water was ingested, but there are many small peaks in the tachygastria frequency, and at the end of the RSA, more peaks at 1 to 2 cpm are seen. This is a pattern of mixed gastric dysrhythmia. The percentage distribution of EGG power graph shows slight increase in tachygastria at baseline and throughout the water load test. The 3-cpm activity is below normal at baseline and remains low at 20 and 30 minutes after ingestion of water. There is a slight increase in bradygastria power at the 30-minute point after ingestion of water. (*B*) EGG with water load test recorded in the same patient approximately 12 months after the radiofrequency ablation procedure for GERD. The RSA shows a series of peaks at 3 cpm at baseline. Water (420 ml) was ingested during the water load test. After the water load, there are clear peaks at 2 cpm, and then a series of lower power peaks at 3 cpm are seen for the remainder of the test. The percentage distribution of EGG power shows the normal baseline and a frequency dip after ingestion of water, which is followed by normal 3-cpm activity 20 and 30 minutes after ingestion of water. There are no bradygastrias. There is a slight increase in tachygastria at 20 and 30 minutes after the ingestion of water. However, overall, this is a normal EGG with a diminished water volume ingested compared with *A*.

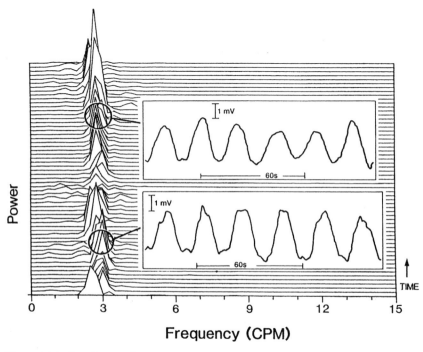

Figure 6.24. Gastric myoelectrical activity in a 59-year-old man with gastric outlet obstruction due to pyloric stenosis. The electrogastrogram (EGG) rhythm strips before and after water load test show high-amplitude regular 3-cpm waves. This patient had documented delayed gastric emptying. The running spectral analysis (RSA) shows unvarying 3-cpm peaks, consistent with obstruction.

Patients with normal gastric electrical rhythm and emptying rates may have visceral hypersensitivity or nongastric causes of their symptoms (category 3). Tricyclic agents such as amitriptyline may help their symptoms. On the other hand, nongastric causes should be considered, and further evaluation of possible GERD (atypical), irritable bowel syndrome, and pancreatic or central nervous system disorders should be considered. These nongastric disorders are treated with specific agents if specific diagnoses are established.

Patients with normal 3-cpm gastric rhythm and gastroparesis are uncommon (category 4). These patients may have electromechanical dissociation or mechanical obstruction. Patients with electromechanical dissociation may respond to bethanechol or erythromycin, which act on the smooth muscle. These drugs may be beneficial because there already is 3-cpm electrical rhythmicity present but enhanced contractility is required. Prokinetic agents may improve electromechanical activity and symptoms, but specific studies are needed in this group of patients. If mechanical obstruction is a possibility, then endoscopy or barium X-ray tests to define the site of obstruction and determine if surgical management is needed. In some cases, pylorospasm or pyloric channel obstructions may be treated by Botox injection or balloon dilatation, respectively.[44]

Patients with chronic nausea and vomiting and gastric neuromuscular dysfunction cannot eat a regular diet. A three-step diet for patients with nausea and vomiting was developed to avoid dehydration (step 1) and to progressively increase the complexity of the diet with liquid (step 2) and solid nutrients (step 3), which require minimal gastric mixing or trituration.[35] The diet is outlined in Table 6.4. Table 6.5 summarizes the four diagnostic categories of gastric neuromuscular disorders based on gastric myoelectrical activity and gastric emptying results. The diagnostic categories and treatments are listed.

Clinical Applications of Electrogastrography in Pediatrics and Obstetrics

EGG methods are useful and safe in clinical evaluation and clinical research involving infants, toddlers, and children. Movement artifacts can be a problem and may limit the duration of the recordings. Normal 3-cpm patterns as well as the gastric dysrhythmia described in

Table 6.4. Diet for Patients with Nausea and Vomiting

Diet	Goal	Avoid
Step 1: Sports Drinks and Bouillon		
For severe nausea and vomiting: • Small volumes of salty liquids, with some caloric content to avoid dehydration • Multiple vitamin	1000–1500 ml/day in multiple servings (e.g., 12 120-ml servings over 12–14 hours) Patient can sip 30–60 ml at a time to reach approximately 120 ml/hr	Citrus drinks of all kinds; highly sweetened drinks
Step 2: Soups		
If sports drink or bouillon tolerated: • Soup with noodles or rice and crackers • Peanut butter, cheese, and crackers in small amounts • Caramels or other chewy confection • Ingest above foods in at least 6 small-volume meals per day • Multiple vitamin	Approximately 1500 calories per day to avoid dehydration and maintain weight (often more realistic than weight gain)	Creamy, milk-based liquids
Step 3: Starches, Chicken, Fish		
If step 2 is tolerated: • Noodles, pastas, potatoes (mashed or baked), rice, baked chicken breast, fish (all easily mixed and emptied by the stomach) • Ingest solids in at least 6 small-volume meals per day • Multiple vitamin	Common foods that patient finds interesting and satisfying and that evoke minimal nausea/vomiting	Fatty foods that delay gastric emptying; red meats and fresh vegetables that require considerable trituration; pulpy fibrous foods that promote formation of bezoars

Source: Modified from Koch KL: Approach to the patient with nausea and vomiting. In: Yamada T, ed. *Textbook of Gastroenterology*, 2nd ed. Philadelphia: JB Lippincott; 1995:731–749.

Table 6.5. Treatment Approaches for Dysmotility-Like Dyspepsia Symptoms Based on Pathophysiological Categories

Category 1: Gastric Dysrhythmia and Gastroparesis	*Category 2: Gastric Dysrhythmia and Normal Emptying*	*Category 3: Normal Gastric Rhythm and Normal Emptying*	*Category 4: Normal Gastric Rhythm and Gastroparesis*
Severe gastric myoelectrocontractile disorder	Gastric myoelectrical disorder	Visceral hypersensitivity* Nongastric causes†	Electrocontractile dissociation* Mechanical obstruction‡
Treatment	*Treatment*	*Treatment*	*Treatment*
Nausea/vomiting diet Prokinetic agents G-tube/J-tube Hyperalimentation Acustimulation Gastric pacemaker	Nausea/vomiting diet Prokinetic agents Antiarrhythmic agents?	Nausea/vomiting diet* Neurosensory agents?* Tricyclic agents* Drugs for fundic compliance?* Further workup for nongastric causes†	Nausea/vomiting diet* Prokinetics* Surgery‡

G-tube, gastrostomy tube; J-tube, jejunostomy tube.

adults have been recorded in infants and children.[45–47] Movement artifacts in the EGG signal are usually high-amplitude, even off-scale signals that are easy to identify. If these signals are digitized and analyzed
by computer, typical artifactual peaks in the Fourier transform or RSA
usually appear.[48] Figure 6.25 is an example of an RSA with two patterns
of artifactual peaks: the "saw-tooth" artifact and the "broad-shoulder"
artifact. When peaks like these are observed, then the original EGG
is reexamined and the EGG signal with artifact is removed from
the minutes of EGG signal that are then resubmitted to computer
analysis.

Another application of EGG is recording gastric myoelectrical
activity from women with nausea of pregnancy. The EGG recording
is safe and provides information on the pathophysiology of nausea in
these women.[9] Figure 6.26 shows gastric dysrhythmias and normal
EGG recordings from women with nausea of pregnancy. Nondrug
treatments of nausea of pregnancy using protein meals[10] and acustimulation[49] represents a novel approach to the diagnosis and treatment of this special condition of nausea.

Applications of Electrogastrography in Research

EGG recordings are used in research studies where changes in gastric myoelectrical activity are a measure of interest. Examples of the
areas the authors have used EGG measures and provocative stimuli
include (1) psychological stressors, (2) motion sickness, cold pressor
tests, and time-shock avoidance stressors, (3) sham feeding, and (4)
mood variables. Other areas related to brain–gut interactions that
incorporate hunger, satiety, and eating disorders have been investigated. Patterns of normal EGG activity, as well as intermittent
bradygastrias and tachygastrias, evolve and develop depending on
different variables in these research protocols.

Summary

The EGG with water load test or other provocative stimuli is a practical clinical test used to measure stomach myoelectrical activity and
gastric capacity. EGG recordings distinguish patients with normal
gastric myoelectrical rhythm from those with gastric dysrhythmias.
Identification of gastric dysrhythmias in adult or pediatric patients

Running Spectral Analysis

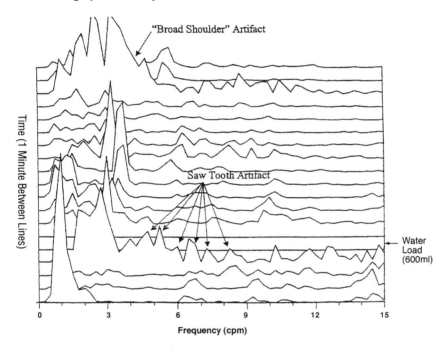

Figure 6.25. Running spectral analysis (RSA) of an electrogastrogram (EGG) with water load test showing artifactual peaks. A "sawtooth" artifact with multiple peaks extending over the 3- to 15-cpm frequencies is shown in the baseline. This artifactual peak suggests a brief movement artifact in the raw EGG signal was included in the minutes submitted for computer analysis. The "broad shoulder" artifact is a high-power peak that extends from 1 to about 6 cpm and is indicated after the water load. This large peak is also produced by movement artifact in the EGG signal. Reexamination of the raw EGG signal is necessary, and the EGG signal containing the artifact is deleted and not included in the computer analysis.

A. Tachygastria

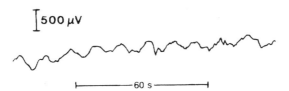

B. Bradygastria (low-amplitude)

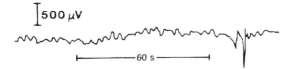

C. Bradygastria (high-amplitude)

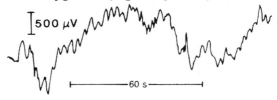

D. Normal

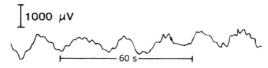

Figure 6.26. Electrogastrogram (EGG) rhythm strips recorded from women with first trimester nausea of pregnancy. A 5- to 6-cpm tachygastria and low-amplitude and high-amplitude bradygastrias are shown. These patients had nausea during the recording, whereas the patient with the normal 3-cpm EGG rhythm had no nausea.

with unexplained dyspepsia symptoms establishes an objective diagnosis, helps the physician to educate the patient regarding the nature of their gastric neuromuscular disorder(s), and directs therapeutic approaches to symptoms based on the pathophysiological abnormalities.

EGG recordings provide objective physiological measures of gastric myoelectrical activity in response to many interesting stimuli. Proper recording techniques, equipment, and interpretation are necessary to avoid misrepresentation and misinterpretation of EGG signal.[48]

The following chapters provide many examples of tachygastrias, bradygastrias, and mixed dysrhythmias recorded from patients with a variety of medical disorders. These chapters are written to assist the clinician and researcher in identifying and interpreting normal and abnormal EGG recordings obtained under controlled, standard conditions.

References

1. Alvarez W: The electrogastrogram and what it shows. *JAMA* 1922;78: 1116–1119.
2. You CH, Lee KY, Chey WY, et al: Electrogastrographic study of patients with unexplained nausea, bloating and vomiting. *Gastroenterology* 1980;79: 311–314.
3. You CH, Chey WY, Lee KY, et al: Gastric and small intestinal myoelectrical dysrhythmia associated with chronic intractable nausea and vomiting. *Ann Intern Med* 1981;95:449–453.
4. Chen JDZ, Schirmer BD, McCallum RW: Serosal and cutaneous recordings of gastric myoelectrical activity in patients with gastroparesis. *Am J Physiol* 1994;266:G90–G98.
5. Smout AJPM, van der Schee EJ, Grashuis JL: What is measured in electrogastrography? *Dig Dis Sci* 1980;25:179–187.
6. Familoni BO, Bowes KL, Kingma YJ, et al: Can transcutaneous recordings detect gastric electrical abnormalities? *Gut* 1991;32:141–146.
7. Stern RM, Koch KL, Leibowitz HW, et al: Tachygastria and motion sickness. Aviat Space Environ Med 1985;56:1074–1077.
8. Stern RM, Koch KL, Stewart WR, et al: Spectral analysis of tachygastria recorded during motion sickness. *Gastroenterology* 1987;92:92–97.
9. Koch KL, Stern RM, Vasey M, et al: Gastric dysrhythmias and nausea of pregnancy. *Dig Dis Sci* 1990;35:961–968.
10. Jednak MA, Shadigian EM, Kim MS, et al: Protein meals reduce nausea and gastric slow wave dysrhythmic activity in first trimester pregnancy. *Am J Physiol* 1999;277:G855–G861.
11. Brzana RJ, Bingaman S, Koch KL: Gastric myoelectrical activity in

patients with gastric outlet obstruction and idiopathic gastroparesis. *Am J Gastroenterol* 1998;93:1083–1089.

12. Koch KL, Stern RM, Stewart WR, et al: Gastric emptying and gastric myoelectrical activity in patients with symptomatic diabetic gastroparesis: effects of long-term domperidone treatment. *Am J Gastroenterol* 1989;84: 1069–1075.

13. Abell TL, Camilleri M, Hench VS, et al: Gastric electromechanical function and gastric emptying in diabetic gastroparesis. *Eur J Gastroenterol Hepatol* 1991; 3:163–167.

14. Jebbink HJA, Bruijs PPM, Varvenboer B, et al: Gastric myoelectrical activity in patients with type I diabetes mellitus and autonomic neuropathy. *Dig Dis Sci* 1994;39:2376–2383.

15. Abell TL, Malagelada J-R: Glucagon-evoked gastric dysrhythmias in humans shown by an improved electrogastrographic technique. *Gastroenterology* 1985;88:1932–1940.

16. Kim CH, Hanson RB, Abell TL, et al: Effect of inhibition of prostaglandin synthesis on epinephrine-induced gastroduodenal electro-mechanical changes in humans. *Mayo Clin Proc* 1989;64:149–157.

17. Kim MS, Chey WD, Owyang C, et al: Role of plasma vasopressin as a mediator of nausea and gastric slow waves dysrhythmias in motion sickness. *Am J Physiol* 1997;G853–G862.

18. Caras SD, Soykian I, Beverly V, et al: The effect of intravenous vasopressin on gastric myoelectrical activity in human subjects. *Neurogastroenterology* 1997;9: 151–156.

19. Kohagen KR, Kim MS, McDonnell WM, et al: Nicotine effects on prostaglandin-dependent gastric slow wave rhythmicity and antral motility in nonsmokers and smokers. *Gastroenterology* 1996;110:3–11.

20. Ladabaum U, Koshy SS, Woods ML, et al: Differential symptomatic and electrogastrographic effects of distal and proximal human gastric distention. *Am J Physiol* 1999;275:G418–G424.

21. Walsh JW, Hasler WL, Nugent CE, et al: Progesterone and estrogen are potential mediators of gastric slow wave dysrhythmias in nausea of pregnancy. *Am J Physiol* 1996;270:G506–G514.

22. Liberski SM, Koch KL, Atnip RG, et al: Ischemic gastroparesis: Resolution after revascularization. *Gastroenterology* 1990;99:252–257.

23. Balaban DH, Chen J, Lin Z, et al: Median arcuate ligament syndrome: possible cause of idiopathic gastroparesis. *Am J Gastroenterol* 1997;92: 519–523.

24. Owyang C, Hasler WL: Physiology and pathophysiology of the interstitial cells of Cajal: from bench to bedside VI pathogenesis and therapeutic approaches to human gastric dysrhythmias. *Am J Physiol* 2002;283: G8–G15.

25. Rothstein RD, Alavai A, Reynolds JC: Electrogastrography in patients with gastroparesis and effect of long-term cisapride. *Dig Dis Sci* 1993;38: 1518–1524.

26. Cucchiara S, Minella R, Riezzo G, et al: Reversal of gastric electrical dysrhythmias by cisapride in children with functional dyspepsia: report of three cases. *Dig Dis Sci* 1992;37:1136–1140.

27. Bersherdas K, Leahy A, Mason I, et al: The effect of cisapride on dyspepsia symptoms and the electrogastrogram in patients with non-ulcer dyspepsia. *Aliment Pharmacol Ther* 1998;12:755–759.

28. Muth ER, Jokerst M, Stern RM, et al: Effects of dimenhydrinate on gastric tachyarrhythmia and symptoms of vection-induced motion sickness. *Aviat Space Environ Med* 1995;66:1041–1045.

29. Hu S, Stern RM, Koch KL: Acustimulation relieves vection-induced motion sickness. *Gastroenterology* 1992;102:1854.

30. McCallum RW, Chen JDZ, Lin ZY, et al: Gastric pacing improves emptying in symptoms in patients with gastroparesis. *Gastroenterology* 1998;114:456–461.

31. Koch KL, Hong S-P, Xu L: Reproducibility of gastric myoelectrical activity and the water load test in patients with dysmotility-like dyspepsia symptoms and in control subjects. *J Clin Gastroenterol* 2000;31:125–129.

32. Parkman HP, Miller MA, Trate D, et al: Electrogastrography in gastric emptying scintigraphy are complimentary for assessment of dyspepsia. *J Clin Gastroenterol* 1997;24:214–219.

33. Talley NJ, Stanghellini V, Heading RC, et al: Functional gastroduodenal disorders. *Gut* 1999;45:1137–1142.

34. Koch KL, Stern RM: Functional disorders of the stomach. *Semin Gastroenterol* 1996;7:185–195.

35. Koch KL: Approach to the patient with nausea and vomiting. In: Yamada T, ed. *Textbook of Gastroenterology*, 2nd ed. Philadelphia: J B Lippincott; 1995:731–749.

36. Stanghellini V, Tosetti C, Paternico A, et al: Risk indicators of delayed gastric emptying of solids in patients with functional dyspepsia. *Gastroenterology* 1996; 110:1038–1042.

37. Lin Z, Eaker EY, Sarosiek I, et al: Gastric myoelectrical activity and gastric emptying in patients with functional dyspepsia. *Am J Gastroenterol* 1999;94:2384–2389.

38. Koch KL: Gastroduodenal motility. In: Brandt LJ, ed. *Clinical Practice in Gastroenterology*. Philadelphia: Current Medicine, Churchill Livingstone; 1998:199–210.

39. Koch KL: Electrogastrography. In: Schuster M, Crowel M, Koch KL, eds. *Atlas of Gastrointestinal Motility*. Hamilton, Ontario, Canada: BC Decker; 2002:185–201.

40. Brzana RJ, Koch KL: Intractable nausea presenting as gastroesophageal reflux disease. *Ann Intern Med* 1997;126:704–707.

41. Koch KL, Xu L, Hong S-P: Spectrum of gastric dysrhythmias and gastric emptying in 54 patients with chronic unexplained nausea and vomiting. *Gastroenterology* 2000;118:A849.

42. Noar M, Koch KL, Xu L: Spectrum of gastric neuromuscular dysfunction in patients with GERD and dysmotility-like functional dyspepsia (GERD+). *Am J Gastroenterol* 2002;122:416A.

43. Stoddard CJ, Smallwood R, Brown BH, et al: The immediate and delayed effects of different types of vagotomy on human gastric myoelectrical activity. *Gut* 1975;16:165–170.

44. Miller LS, Szych GA, Kantor SB, et al: Treatment of idiopathic gastroparesis with injection of Botulinum toxin into the pyloric sphincter muscle. *Am J Gastroenterol* 2002;97:1653–1660.

45. Koch KL, Tran T, Bingaman S, et al: Gastric myoelectrical activity in fasted and fed premature and term infants. *J Gastrointestin Motil* 1993;5: 41–47.

46. Cucchiara S, Salvia G, Scarcella A, et al: Gestational maturation of electrical activity of the stomach. *Dig Dis Sci* 1999;44:2008–2013.

47. Liang J, Co E, Zhang M, et al: Development of gastric slow waves in preterm infants measured by electrogastrography. *Am J Physiol* 1998;274: G503–G508.

48. Verhagen MAMT, VanSchelven CJ, Samson M, et al: Pitfalls in the analysis of electrogastrographic recordings. *Gastroenterology* 1999;117:453–460.

49. Evans A, Sammuels S, Marshall C, et al: Suppression of pregnancy induced nausea and vomiting with sensory afferent stimulation. *J Reprod Med* 1993; 8:603–606.

7

Tachygastrias

Gastric dysrhythmias are abnormal myoelectrical signals originating from the stomach. As recorded from cutaneous or
serosal electrodes, bradygastrias range from 0 to 2.5 cycles
per minute (cpm).[1-8] Bradygastrias and mixed gastric dysrhythmias
are reviewed in detail in Chapter 8. Tachygastrias range from 3.75 to
10.0 cpm.[1,5,6,8-12] The normal duodenal pacesetter potential ranges
from 12 to 14 cpm.[13] In this chapter, tachygastrias are reviewed in
detail.

Pathophysiology of Gastric Dysrhythmias

Multiple metabolic mechanisms and neural-hormonal pathways influence gastric myoelectrical activity. The normal activities of enteric neurons, smooth muscle, hormones, and extrinsic nerves influence the
ongoing activity of the interstitial cells of Cajal (ICCs), the pacemaker
cells of the stomach.[14-16] In healthy subjects, the frequency of gastric myoelectrical activity may vary from approximately 2.5 to 3.7 cpm, depending on specific circumstances or provocative tests[1,2,17] (Fig. 7.1).
Specific diseases and disorders, with their specific pathophysiologies,

149

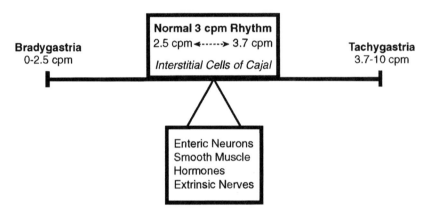

Figure 7.1. Normal gastric myoelectrical rhythm and gastric dysrhythmias. The normal 3-cpm electrogastrographic rhythm ranges from 2.5 to 3.7 cpm and reflects gastric pacesetter potentials that are produced by the interstitial cells of Cajal (ICCs). ICC activity is modulated by activities of the enteric neurons, smooth muscle cells, the extrinsic parasympathetic and sympathetic nervous systems, and hormones. Transient shifts from normal 3-cpm rhythm to bradygastrias (0–2.5 cpm) and tachygastrias (3.7–10 cpm) can occur in healthy patients. Patients with a variety of diseases and disorders have persistent, clinically relevant bradygastrias and tachygastrias.

may adversely affect gastric myoelectrical activity and are associated with gastric dysrhythmias. For example, many patients with type I and II diabetes have gastric dysrhythmias,[18,19] and in healthy subjects, hyperglycemia itself produces gastric dysrhythmias.[20]

Gastric dysrhythmias occur when the ICCs are damaged or dysfunctional or when enteric neurons, circular smooth muscle cells (and perhaps longitudinal muscle activity), and extrinsic nerve activity from the parasympathetic and sympathetic nervous system input to the stomach are abnormal. Endocrine, neurocrine, and paracrine activities may also affect interstitial cells, enteric neurons, and smooth muscle and thereby affect gastric myoelectrical rhythms,[21] shifting electrical activity to bradygastrias (0–2.5 cpm) or tachygastrias (3.7–10.0 cpm) as shown in Figure 7.1. All of these influences interact to maintain normal gastric myoelectrical activity during baseline periods and in response to meals or other provocative stimuli. Stimuli that provoke stomach neuromuscular activity range from motion and the illusion of motion to emotionally challenging situations (disgust, anger) to the cephalic phase of digestion (vagal activation in the presence of appetizing food) to the relaxation, contraction, and coordination of stomach neuromuscular responses during and after the ingestion of a wide variety of solid and liquid foodstuffs. Thus, there are many gut–brain and brain–gut interactions to consider when evaluating gastric myoelectrical events during EGG recordings at baseline and after provocative stimuli.

Origin of Tachygastrias

Knowledge of the basic mechanisms of gastric dysrhythmias in humans is advancing. Tachygastrias have been induced in various studies, which suggest specific underlying mechanisms. Vagotomy results in the onset of tachygastria, findings that suggest sympathetic nervous system "dominance" evokes tachygastrias.[2,22] Epinephrine infusions induced tachygastrias.[23] The percentage of EGG power in the tachygastria range correlated significantly with plasma epinephrine in healthy subjects who experienced nausea during motion sickness.[24] Furthermore, withdrawal of vagal tone and increased sympathetic tone as measured by respiratory sinus arrhythmia and skin conductance are associated with tachygastrias and motion sickness.[25] Taken together, these data suggest that loss of vagal parasympathetic activity and/or increase in sympathetic nervous system activity evokes tachy-gastrias. The shift in gastric myoelectrical rhythm from the normal 3-cpm frequency to tachygastria or bradygastria may alter vagal (or sympathetic) afferent nerve activity, which initiates the perception of noxious visceral sensations.[26]

Glucagon, nicotine, estrogens and progesterones, and hyper-glycemia evoke gastric dysrhythmias and nausea symptoms in humans,[9,19,27,28] indicating multiple pathways can disrupt normal gastric myoelectrical activity. The hyperglycemia-induced dysrhythmias are reduced by pretreatment with indomethacin and indicates a key role of prostaglandins in the mechanism of these gastric dysrhythmias.[19] Thus, a variety of receptors on nerve, smooth muscle are relevant to gastric dysrhythmias in certain patients or certain research conditions.

From a cellular viewpoint, dysfunction of the ICCs may result in bradygastrias or tachygastrias. Knockout mice (W/W^v) with decreased or absent ICCs have increased gastric dysrhythmias, contraction abnormalities and decreased transit of intraluminal contents compared with wild-type mice.[15,16,29] Prostaglandin E appears to have a role in controlling pacesetter potential frequency, possibly by influencing the frequency of ICC depolarization/repolarization.[29,30] Intrinsic inhibitory or excitatory neurons influence the electrical rhythmicity of the ICCs and lead to transient nonpathological dysrhythmias or to permanent dysrhythmias in disease states. In some cases, the smooth muscle itself may be irritable and result in rapid and irregular contractions that are in the 3.7 to 10 per minute range.[31]

The presence of gastric dysrhythmias may affect vagal (and possibly splanchnic) afferent nerve activity.[26] Figure 7.2 shows visceral and somatic nerve connections between the stomach and central nervous system (CNS) through the vagus nerve and the spinal cord. Vagal afferent impulses are transmitted to the nucleus tractus solitarius and higher CNS centers where symptoms such as nausea are recognized and experienced. Splanchnic afferent activity is transmitted through the dorsal horn cells of the spinal cord and then to CNS centers.

Somatic afferent nerves carry C and A delta fibers from the skin, for example, to the dorsal horn cells of the spinal cord where afferent sensory information is transferred to the central nervous system and perceived as pleasant or noxious somatic sensations. On the

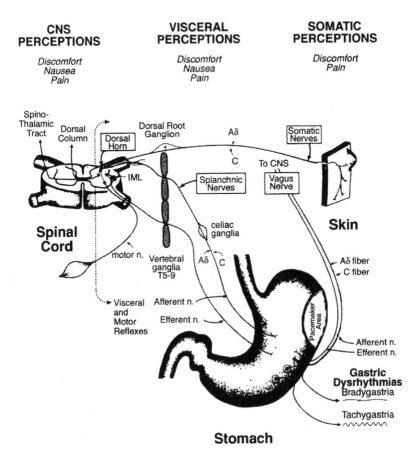

CNS PERCEPTIONS	VISCERAL PERCEPTIONS	SOMATIC PERCEPTIONS
Discomfort *Nausea* *Pain*	*Discomfort* *Nausea* *Pain*	*Discomfort* *Pain*

Figure 7.2. Pathways from the gastric visceral nervous systems and the somatic nervous system (skin) to the spinal cord are shown. Gastric neuromuscular disorders range from abnormalities of fundic tone to gastric dysrhythmias and abnormalities of relaxation and contraction of the muscular wall. These peripheral neuromuscular events in the stomach may alter vagal or splanchnic afferent nerve activity. Purely afferent nerve abnormalities may also be present and result in hypersensitivity. The sympathetic afferent impulses (C fibers and Aδ fibers) are transmitted to the brain via synapses in the dorsal horn cells and the dorsal column and spinothalamic tracts. Perceptions of epigastric discomfort, pain and nausea are identified in the cortex. Somatic nerves containing C fibers transmit noxious stimuli to the dorsal horn cells and then through the spinothalamic tracts to the central nervous system where localized somatic pain is identified.

153

other hand, afferent nerve activity from the viscera pass into the CNS via vagal or splanchnic afferent pathways. Splanchnic nerve fibers pass through the vertebral ganglia and then proceed to the dorsal horn cells and ascend to CNS pathways, where visceral discomfort, nausea, and pain are perceived. Efferent motor pathways for the visceral and somatic systems are also shown.

CNS activity may also influence gastric neuromuscular function via parasympathetic and sympathetic nervous system efferent pathways and the release of stress hormones such as adrenocorticotropin hormone, cortisol, and vasopressin, which may also affect gastric neuromuscular activity.[24] As shown in Figure 7.3, the relevant anatomical areas for vagal afferent nerve activity includes the nucleus tractus solitarius, area postrema, hypothalamus, limbic region, and areas of the cortex where nausea and bloating sensations are perceived. The transition from eugastria to tachygastria that occurs during motion sickness is shown in Figure 7.3. During and after this shift in gastric rhythm, increased vasopressin, epinephrine, and cortisol are released into plasma[24] (Fig. 7.3). Thus, gut–brain and brain–gut interactions occur during the development of noxious visceral sensations such as nausea. Many other cognitive and emotional stimuli result in altered gastric myoelectrical responses, such as the altered EGG response to sham feeding in subjects who considered the sham feeding "disgusting."

The complexity of the gastric neuromuscular apparatus also underscores the importance of standard and straightforward provocative testing when the EGG rhythm pattern is assessed in research or clinical situations. In later sections, examples of tachygastria and poor 3-cpm response to the water load test are shown. EGG rhythm strips, running spectral analysis (RSA), and percentage distribution of the EGG power in four relevant frequency ranges are depicted in the figures. Analysis of these records is the basis for the clinical diagnosis of normal myoelectrical rhythm or gastric dysrhythmias. Other test meals or other provocative stimuli may be used to evoke symptoms or changes in EGG rhythm depending on the objectives of the testing. The tachygastria, bradygastria, and mixed dysrhythmia patterns are the same regardless of the subject or the recording situation.

Examples of normal 3-cpm EGG activity, tachygastria, and bradygastria are shown in Figures 7.4, 7.5, and 7.6. Each figure shows a 4-minute EGG rhythm strip. Below the EGG rhythm strip is the Fourier transform for those 4 minutes of EGG signal. The Fourier

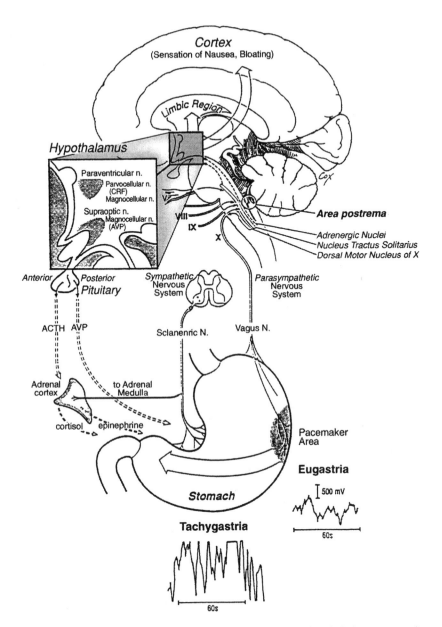

Figure 7.3. Brain–gut and gut–brain interactions during the shift from eugastria to tachygastria. Vagal and splanchnic nervous systems connect with central nervous system structures such as the hypothalamus, area postrema, and cortex, areas that are relevant for the perception of visceral sensations such as nausea and bloating. Neural efferent activity from the parasympathetic and sympathetic nervous systems or stress hormones such as epinephrine, cortisol, and vasopressin (AVP) may alter gastric neuromuscular activity such as the pacesetter potentials.

155

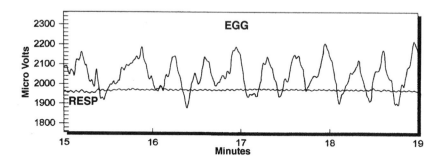

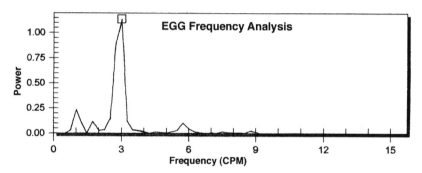

Figure 7.4. A 4-minute electrogastrogram (EGG) rhythm strip (minutes 15–19) is shown in the *top panel.* Respiration (RESP) signal is also shown running through the EGG waves. The EGG frequency analysis by Fourier transform (FT) is shown in the *bottom panel.* The EGG rhythm strip shows 3-cpm EGG waves. The FT calculates the frequencies that occur within the 4-minute EGG signal. Power is a unitless number that indicates the strengths of any frequencies contained in the 4-minute EGG signal. As shown in the frequency analysis, the highest peak (and power) is located at the frequency of 3 cpm, a frequency consistent with the regular 3 cpm EGG waves shown in the EGG signal. The small peak at 6 cpm represents a harmonic of the primary 3-cpm frequency.

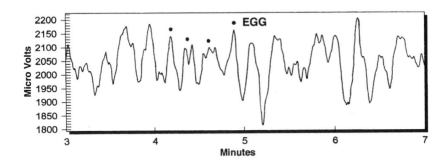

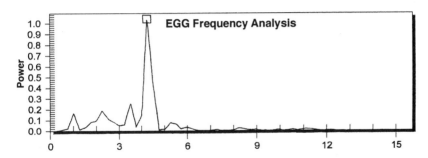

Figure 7.5. The electrogastrogram (EGG) signal (*top panel*) shows a tachygastria with a frequency of approximately 4 cpm. The black dots indicate the 4-cpm tachygastria waves during minute 4 of the recording. EGG waves at 4 to 5 cpm are also present in minutes 3 to 7 of the recording. The EGG frequency analysis (*bottom panel*) by FT shows the highest peak (power) is approximately 4 cpm, an abnormally fast frequency in the tachygastria range that is consistent with the 4-cpm EGG waves. There are low power peaks in the lower frequencies (1–2 cpm). Overall, the EGG signal and FT frequency analysis indicates a tachygastria at approximately 4 cpm.

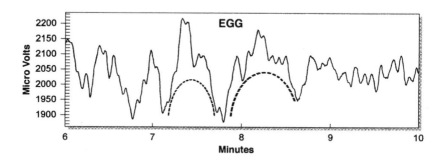

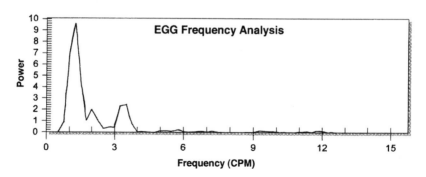

Figure 7.6. The electrogastrogram (EGG) rhythm strip in the top panel shows large amplitude waves at approximately 1 cpm in minutes 6, 7, and 8. The dotted lines under the EGG waves in minutes 7 and 8 indicate the 1 cpm EGG waves. The EGG Frequency Analysis (lower panel) shows the highest peak (power) is at the 1–1.5 cpm frequency, consistent with the frequency seen in the EGG signal.

transform computes the frequencies that are contained in the 4 minutes of EGG signal, as discussed in Chapter 5. In the present examples, the EGG rhythm strips clearly show 3-, 4-, and 2-cpm EGG waves, respectively. The large peak in the Fourier transform beneath each EGG rhythm strip indicates that the frequency in the EGG signal is a consistent 3-cpm (normal), a 4-cpm rhythm (tachygastria), or a 2-cpm (bradygastria) frequency, respectively. The peaks in the Fourier transforms indicate the power at the various frequencies contained in the EGG signal. The power is the log of the microvolt squared as calculated from the raw EGG signal. Thus, the Fourier transform is an objective measure of the power of the frequencies contained in EGG signals.

Tachygastrias

The EGGs shown in these figures were recorded from patients with unexplained nausea or dyspepsia symptoms. The tracings are from a 15-minute baseline recording and the 30 minutes after the water load test. The water load test is a provocative test of stomach distention (relaxation), followed by electrical and contractile activity of the stomach that is elicited to empty the volume of water into the duodenum. The patient or volunteer fasts after midnight and then eats one piece of unbuttered toast and drinks 4 oz. of apple juice 2 hours before the EGG test. The breakfast snack is standardized to ensure a consistent baseline EGG.[17] This light snack of approximately 200 calories prevents severe hunger (and sometimes nausea) and prevents phase III contractions that may occur during prolonged fasting. The subject then fasts for 2 hours after the snack until the water load test is performed. Details of the water load test protocol are described in Chapter 6.

Tachygastria includes frequencies from 3.75 to 10.0 cpm. For purposes of presentation, the tachygastrias are divided into "unifocal" tachygastrias because there is a single predominant tachygastria frequency recorded in the EGG (e.g., 4-cpm tachygastrias, as shown in Fig. 7.5). In contrast, the diffuse or multifocal tachygastria is a pattern with multiple frequencies in the tachygastria range. When either the unifocal or diffuse tachygastria pattern is present, there usually is poor 3-cpm EGG activity. "Probable tachygastrias" are described when normal 3-cpm activity is present, but the tachygastrias are intermittently seen in the raw EGG signal, in the running spectral analyses (RSAs), and in the percentage distribution of EGG power analyses. Harmonics and artifacts must be excluded as potential sources of the tachygastria peaks in the RSA.

Tachygastrias (Unifocal)

A very clear unifocal tachygastria at 4 cpm is shown first. Figure 7.7 shows the EGG rhythm strips, the RSA, and percentage distribution of EGG power from an elderly woman with chronic nausea. A 4-cpm tachygastria is seen in the EGG rhythm strips (A and B) in Figure 7.7. The analysis of this EGG—the EGG rhythm strip, the RSA, and the percentage distribution of EGG power—is described in detail. Other figures in this chapter are presented in a similar format and are not described in as much detail. The EGG rhythm strips (A and B) in Figure 7.7 are selected from baseline and after water load portions of the EGG and water load test. At baseline, a 4-cpm EGG signal is seen (A). The 4 cpm EGG signal persists after ingestion of water (B).

The RSA in Figure 7.7 shows frequencies in cycles per minute from 0 to 15 cpm on the X-axis. The Y-axis indicates time, with each line representing 4 minutes of EGG signal with a 75% overlap. Thus, each new line represents 1 minute of new EGG data added to the previous 3 minutes. The Z-axis indicates the power of the signal at whatever frequencies are contained in the EGG signal. Strong frequencies in the EGG signal appears as higher peaks at those same frequencies in the RSA. The RSA from the baseline period shows peaks at approximately 4.5 cpm (A1), with little or no peaks in the normal 3-cpm range. The water load volume was 400 ml and is indicated by the arrow and the two flat lines in the RSA. Healthy subjects ingest 600 ml of water in 5 minutes on average.[17] After ingestion of the water load, there was temporary suppression of the 4-cpm activity as shown by the loss of 4-cpm peaks. The RSA peaks at B1 show that the 4-cpm EGG activity returned. The RSA peaks at 4-cpm reflect the 4-cpm tachygastria waves shown in the EGG rhythm strips.

The percentage distribution of EGG power shows the percentage of all of the EGG power from 0 to 15 cpm in the four relevant frequency ranges: bradygastria, normal, tachygastria, and duodenal respiration. The percentages from 0% to 100% are presented on the Y-axis. Baseline (BL) and 10, 20, and 30 minutes after ingestion of water are the time points on the X-axis. The solid dark line represents

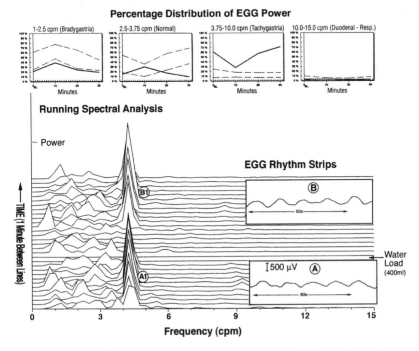

Figure 7.7. Tachygastria with abnormal water load test. This figure shows electrogastrogram (EGG) rhythm strips before (*A*) and after (*B*) a water load, the running spectral analysis (RSA) of the EGG signal before and after the water load, and the percentage distribution of EGG power in the four relevant frequency ranges at baseline (BL) and 10, 20, and 30 minutes after the water load. These components are described in detail in the text. The EGG rhythm strips show a 4-cpm tachygastria. The RSA shows peaks at 4 cpm before and after the 400 ml water load. The percentage distribution of EGG power shows increased tachygastria and a poor 3-cpm response to the water load. The raw EGG and quantitative analyses of the EGG are reviewed to establish an overall clinical EGG diagnosis. In this case, the diagnosis is tachygastria with an abnormal water load test. Other figures in this chapter are presented in a similar format.

this patient's percentage distribution of EGG power, whereas the dashed lines indicate the mean ± 1 SD of EGG power recorded from healthy subjects who underwent the water load test. Figures 3.13, 3.14, and 3.15 show the normal EGG response to water load test in healthy subjects and are helpful comparisons with the tachygastrias shown here. In this patient, the distribution of EGG power in the bradygastria range was low, the normal EGG activity was low at baseline and then increased into the normal range 10 minutes after water was ingested, but then declined to below normal activity 20 and 30 minutes after the water load. On the other hand, the tachygastria power was elevated at baseline. Tachygastria power decreased during the 10 minutes after ingestion of water but then increased 20 and 30 minutes after the ingestion of the water. The duodenal-respiratory percentage was within normal limits. Thus, the increased percentage distribution of EGG power in the tachygastria range reflects the many 4- to 5-cpm peaks present in the RSA, which reflects the 4-cpm waves in the raw EGG signal. The clinical diagnosis is tachygastria and poor water load volume.

Another unifocal tachygastria is shown in Figure 7.8, but more variability in the tachygastria is present compared with Figure 7.7. The EGG rhythm strip from baseline (A) in Figure 7.8 show a 5- to 6-cpm tachygastria in a middle-aged woman with nausea and vomiting. The 5- to 6-cpm tachygastria persists in the EGG rhythm strips after the water load test (B). The RSA during baseline shows the highest peaks are at the 5- to 6-cpm frequency (A1), consistent with the frequencies seen in the EGG signal. The patient ingested 750 ml, which is a normal volume, during the 5-minute water load test. After ingestion of water, a few 3-cpm peaks in the RSA increase briefly in the first 10 minutes but do not increase thereafter. On the other hand, peaks in the RSA persist in the 5- to 6-cpm tachygastria frequency (B1), as also seen in the EGG rhythm strip (B). The percentage distribution of EGG power graphs show low percentage of power in the bradygastria range throughout the test. The normal 3-cpm EGG activity increases slightly at 10 minutes after the ingestion of water and then remains below normal 20 and 30 minutes thereafter. The tachygastria percentages are elevated before and 10, 20, and 30 minutes after the water load test. Thus, the stomach had a normal capacity for the water load, but the gastric electrical pattern after the water load was a persistent tachygastria at 5 to 6 cpm.

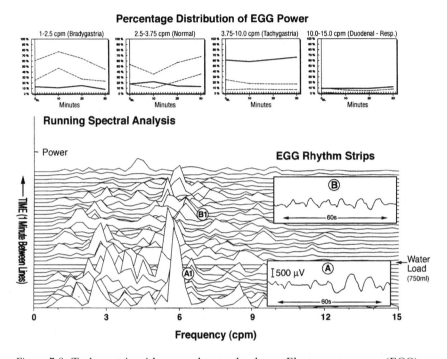

Percentage Distribution of EGG Power

Figure 7.8. Tachygastria with normal water load test. Electrogastrogram (EGG) rhythm strips, running spectral analysis (RSA), and percentage distribution of EGG power are shown in a patient with chronic nausea and vomiting. The format of the figure is the same as Figure 7.7. The baseline EGG rhythm strip (*A*) shows a 5- to 6-cpm EGG rhythm that persists (*B*) after the water load. The RSA during baseline also shows the highest peaks are at the 5- to 6-cpm frequency (A1). After the ingestion of water, 3-cpm peaks in the RSA appear in the first 10 minutes, but thereafter, peaks in the RSA persist at the 5- to 6-cpm tachygastria frequency (B1). The percentage distribution of EGG power graphs show a low percentage of power in the bradygastria range. The percentage of normal 3-cpm EGG activity increases 10 minutes after ingestion of water but then decreases below normal at 20 and 30 minutes. The tachygastria percentages are elevated before and 10, 20, and 30 minutes after the water load test. Thus, this is a 5- to 6-cpm tachygastria with a normal water load test.

A unifocal tachygastria at approximately 7 to 8 cpm recorded from a college student with chronic nausea and gastroparesis after a viral illness is shown in Figure 7.9. The EGG rhythm strips show the 7- to 8-cpm tachygastria very clearly before (A) and after (B) ingestion of water. This patient ingested very little water (250 ml) and "felt full." At baseline, the RSA shows peaks in the 7- to 8-cpm range (A1) and very small 3-cpm peaks. After ingestion of 250 ml of water, several peaks at 3 cpm are seen initially and then disappear. Peaks at 8-cpm reappear in the remainder of the RSA (B1) and reflect the 8-cpm tachygastria in the EGG signal (B). The EGG activity is reflected in a quantitative fashion in the percentage distribution of EGG power graphs. The bradygastria percentages are low throughout the test. A brief increase in the percentage of 3-cpm activity is seen at 10 minutes after ingestion of water, but then decrease below normal at 20 and 30 minutes. On the other hand, the percentage of tachygastria power is increased at baseline, decreases 10 minutes after ingestion of water, but then increases at 20 and 30 minutes. The EGG diagnosis is tachygastria with abnormal water load test.

Distention of the fasted antrum and corpus requires relaxation of the smooth muscle of the stomach (see Fig. 3.10). Normal relaxation of the stomach reduces wall tension in response to ingestion of volumes of solid and liquid meals. Patients with unexplained dyspepsia symptoms drink significantly less water or caloric meals compared with healthy control subjects.[17,32,33] The ingestion of water frequently evokes nausea and bloating symptoms.[17] Gastric dysrhythmias may or may not be elicited by distending of the stomach walls during water loading in these patients. If stomach fullness is perceived but only small volumes of water are consumed, then decreased gastric capacity and decreased ability of the stomach to relax and receive the volume are indicated.

The potential gastric myoelectrical responses to a water load test in a patient with unexplained nausea and dyspepsia symptoms are illustrated in Figure 7.10. Gastric myoelectrical activity at the normal 3-cpm pattern is recorded during the fasting EGG, and the 3-cpm myoelectrical activity is also recorded by the serosal electrodes. Fasting volume of the normal stomach is approximately 50 ml.[34] The patient in this example ingested only 250 ml of water and felt full. Two gastric myoelectrical responses are shown. The post water load EGG signal at A shows a normal 3-cpm signal, and the serosal signal A also shows a 3-cpm signal after the water load. Thus, in some

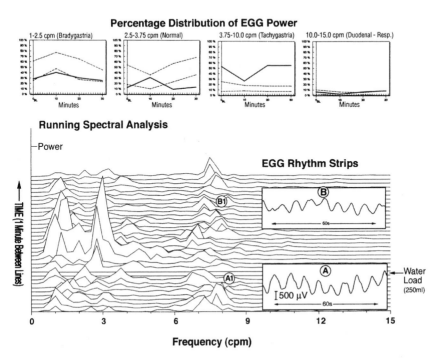

Percentage Distribution of EGG Power

1-2.5 cpm (Bradygastria)   2.5-3.75 cpm (Normal)   3.75-10.0 cpm (Tachygastria)   10.0-15.0 cpm (Duodenal - Resp.)

Minutes   Minutes   Minutes   Minutes

Running Spectral Analysis

Power

EGG Rhythm Strips

TIME (1 Minute Between Lines)

B1

B

60s

A1

A

500 µV

60s

Water
Load
(250ml)

0   3   6   9   12   15

Frequency (cpm)

Figure 7.9. Tachygastria with poor water load test in a college student with chronic nausea. The format is similar to Figure 7.7. The electrogastrogram (EGG) rhythm strips (A and B) show 8-cpm tachygastrias before and after the water load. The running spectral analysis (RSA) shows peaks in the 7- to 8-cpm range (A1) at baseline and very little 3-cpm peaks. After ingestion of 250 ml of water, several peaks at 3 cpm are seen initially and then disappear. The 8-cpm peaks reappear in the later minutes of the RSA (B1) and reflect the 8-cpm tachygastria (B). The EGG activity is reflected in a quantitative fashion in the percentage distribution of EGG power graphs. A brief increase in the percentage of 3-cpm activity is seen at 10 minutes after ingestion of water, but 3-cpm percentages decrease below normal 20 and 30 minutes after ingestion. On the other hand, the percentage of power in the tachygastria range is increased at baseline, decreases 10 minutes

Patient with Nausea
(250 ml)

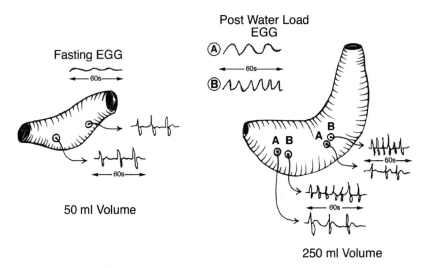

Figure 7.10. Illustration of the stomach during fasting and after a patient ingests water until full. In this example, the fasting stomach volume is 50 ml. Normal 3-cpm myoelectrical activity is recorded from serosal electrodes and the normal 3-cpm electrogastrographic signal is present. After the stomach is distended physically with the 250 ml of water ingested during the water load test, the stomach either remains in a normal 3-cpm rhythm (A) or converts to tachygastria (B) as shown by the serosal electrode recordings (A) and (B) or the post water load EGG signals at A and B. (As discussed in Chapter 8, bradygastrias or mixed dysrhythmias may also develop after ingestion of food or water.)

patients, the water load does not evoke a shift from the normal 3-cpm rhythm. The post water load EGG signal B, however, shows a tachygastria evoked during the water load. The tachygastria is also illustrated by the serosal recording (B). In patients with GERD plus dyspepsia symptoms, the provocative water loading test unmasked approximately 40% more gastric dysrhythmias compared with baseline.[35] Thus, stretch of the antrum produced by the water load may evoke gastric dysrhythmias.

Tachygastrias may appear at any frequency from 3.7 to 10.0 cpm. Figure 7.11 shows a unifocal tachygastria at approximately 10 cpm that was brought on after the 739-ml water load. The baseline EGG rhythm strip (A) shows a variety of frequencies with 1 to 2 cpm and other frequencies as well, such as 8 to 9 cpm. This is an unstable fasting EGG signal. The RSA from the baseline period also shows peaks ranging from 1 to 2 cpm to 5 to 6 cpm (A1) to 9 to 10 cpm. There are very few 3-cpm peaks in the RSA during baseline. After ingestion of the water, few 3-cpm peaks developed in the RSA. An increase in peaks in the 1-to 2-cpm frequency is seen. There are clear peaks in the RSA at approximately 9 to 10 cpm (B1) and (C1) after the water load. The EGG rhythm strips at B and C show the 9- to 10-cpm tachygastrias, which are clearly the prominent pattern in the raw EGG signal. Figure 7.11C shows the 9-cpm tachygastria with the simultaneous respiration recording. The respirations rate is 18 per minute. Thus, the 9- to 10-cpm EGG activity is clearly not a respiratory rhythm. The percentage distribution of EGG power graphs show bradygastria activity is within the normal range. (Peaks at 1 to 2 cpm are seen in the RSA, but the overall percentage of power in the bradygastria range is within the normal range.) The 3-cpm EGG power is very low throughout the recording. The percentage of EGG activity in the tachygastria range is persistently elevated. Thus, the clinical EGG interpretation is a tachygastria with normal water load test.

These tachygastrias are termed as "unifocal" for descriptive purposes only. The origins of unifocal tachygastrias are not known. Unifocal tachygastrias have been recorded from the antrum in canine and human studies using serosal electrodes. The unifocal tachygastria suggests there is a single irritable focus, possibly within the ICCs, that is spontaneously depolarizing and repolarizing at regular but abnormal tachygastria frequencies. The irritable focus of cells entrains other cells to oscillate at the abnormal frequency. Injury to or dysfunction of intrinsic inhibitory (or excitatory) neurons may also have a role in the

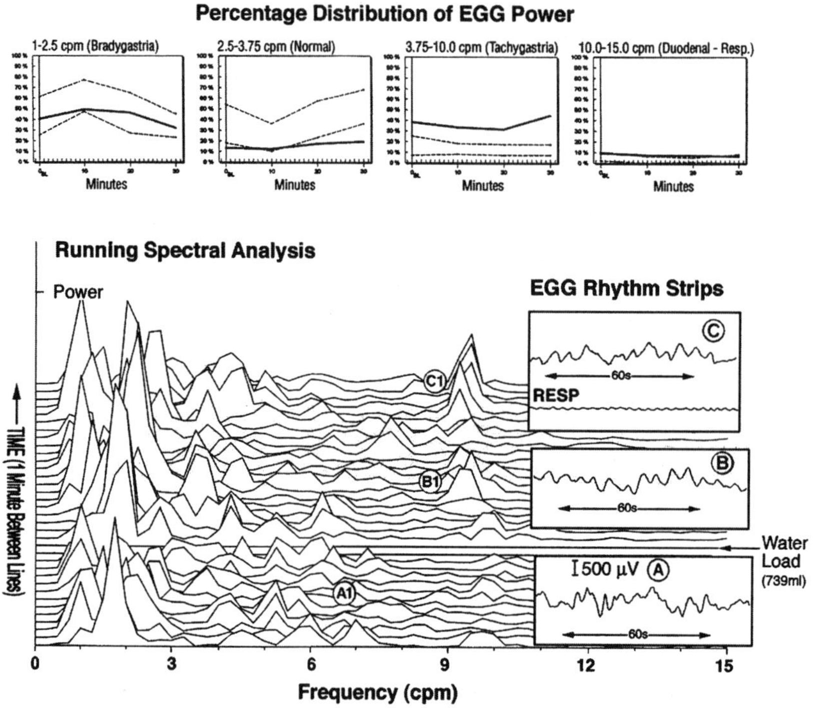

Percentage Distribution of EGG Power

Figure 7.11. Tachygastria with normal water load test. Electrogastrogram (EGG) rhythm strips, running spectral analysis (RSA), and percentage distribution of EGG power from a patient with idiopathic chronic nausea. The baseline EGG rhythm strip (A) shows a variety of frequencies with 1 to 2 cpm and other frequencies as well, e.g., 7 to 9 cpm. The RSA from the baseline also shows frequency peaks ranging from 1 to 2 cpm to 5 to 7 cpm (A1) to 9 to 10 cpm. Very small 3-cpm peaks are present. After the water load, there are few 3-cpm peaks in the RSA and an increase in peaks in the 1- to 2-cpm activity. There are clear peaks in the RSA at approximately 9 to 10 cpm (B1 and C1). The EGG rhythm strips at B and C show 9- to 10-cpm tachygastrias. C depicts the 9-cpm EGG activity with the simultaneous respiration recording indicating the breathing rate is 18 per minute. The percentage distribution of EGG power graphs shows normal bradygastria activity during the test. The percentage of 3-cpm EGG power is very low, and the percentage of EGG activity in the tachygastria range is persistently elevated. Thus, the clinical EGG interpretation is tachygastria with normal water load test.

generation of the unifocal tachygastrias. It is unlikely that unifocal tachygastrias originate from smooth muscle because gastric myopathies are associated with very irregular, chaotic EGG frequencies.[31]

Tachygastrias have been recorded after vagotomy and epinephrine infusion,[2,22,23] suggesting "sympathetic nervous system dominance" has a role in the pathogenesis of the tachygastrias. Other mechanisms may mediate tachygastrias, because nicotine,[27] glucagon,[9] and hyperglycemia[19] also induce tachygastrias. Kohagen et al. found nicotine-induced dysrhythmias are not mediated by prostaglandins,[27] whereas hyperglycemia-induced dysrhythmias are mediated by prostaglandin pathways because pretreatment with indomethacin prevented these dysrhythmias.[20] In animal studies, prostaglandin E_2 increased pacesetter potential frequency and indomethacin decreased pacesetter potential frequency.[30] Tachygastria rhythms may be stationary or be propagated orally or aborally. As described in Figure 6.8, the presence of tachygastrias in humans is associated with greater delays in gastric emptying compared with bradygastrias. In the next section, tachygastrias with more erratic frequencies are shown. For descriptive reasons, these tachygastrias are termed *diffuse tachygastrias*.

Tachygastrias (Diffuse)

Tachygastrias may continually vary in frequency from 3.7 to 10.0 cpm during the recording period. These varying frequencies are seen in the EGG signal and in the varying peaks at different tachygastria frequencies in the RSA. For example, frequencies in the raw EGG signal may vary minute by minute from 4 to 5 to 7 cpm, and visual inspection of the EGGs reveals very little normal 3-cpm activity.

The EGG signal is the summation of the myoelectrical frequencies that are occurring on the stomach beneath the recording electrodes positioned on the epigastrium. Two or more tachygastrias of different frequency may occur independently,[36] a type of multifocal tachygastria. Or, a single focus of myoelectrical irritability in the antrum corpus may be constantly changing in frequency and thereby produce an irregular pattern of tachygastria, that is, a diffuse tachygastria to distinguish this pattern from the unifocal tachygastria.

The concept of "uncoupling" has been described in experiments in dog.[37] The neuromuscular wall of the stomach was divided by surgical incision, rendering one area "uncoupled" electrically from the distal part of the stomach. ICC networks, enteric nervous system connections, and smooth muscle cells were disrupted by the incision of the gastric wall. In this postsurgical situation, two or more distinct gastric electrical frequencies were present at the same time on the surface of the stomach.[37] (In this setting, the antrum reverted to a slower "normal intrinsic" pacesetter potential frequency of 1 to 2 cpm, an observation that is relevant to origins of bradygastrias described in the next chapter.) From the cutaneous EGG recordings, different myoelectrical frequencies occurring simultaneously in the stomach are "summed" and the result is an abnormal EGG—a gastric dysrhythmia with an overall pattern of tachygastria, bradygastria, or mixed dysrhythmia.

An example of a diffuse tachygastria is shown in Figure 7.12. The EGG rhythm strip (A) from baseline shows broad, long-duration waves that are bradygastrias, but there are also low-amplitude faster frequencies in the baseline EGG signal. The RSA also shows a variety of peaks during baseline, including peaks from 2.5 to 3.7 cpm (A1) and some peaks in the 1- to 2-cpm range. This patient ingested 296 ml of water during the water load, an abnormally low volume. There was very little 3-cpm EGG activity in (B) and (C). After ingestion of water, the frequencies in the EGG rhythm strips vary from approximately 8 cpm as shown in (B) to 5 cpm as shown in (C). These tachygastria frequencies are also reflected in the RSA at (B1) (see small peaks at 8 cpm) and (C1) (see peaks at 5 to 6 cpm). Thus, in comparison to the tachygastrias in Figures 7.7, 7.8, and 7.9, this EGG has more variable tachygastria frequencies (i.e., diffuse pattern). There are peaks in the bradygastria range in the RSA, but the overall percentages of power in the bradygastria ranges are within the normal range or lower. The percentage distribution of EGG power in the normal 3-cpm range decreases throughout the post water load time period, whereas while the tachygastria percentage increases 10, 20, and 30 minutes after the water load. The water load shifted the normal baseline EGG pattern to a tachygastria pattern in this patient. Thus, the clinical interpretation is tachygastria with abnormal water load test.

In some patients, the tachygastria erupts in a high-amplitude dysrhythmia that is similar to the acute tachygastrias recorded during motion sickness. Figure 7.13 shows a tachygastria, diffuse pattern that developed after the water load. The baseline EGG had multiple frequencies in the EGG rhythm strip (A). The patient ingested only 250 ml of water during the water load test. The EGG rhythm strip B shows a prominent 4-cpm tachygastria that developed toward the

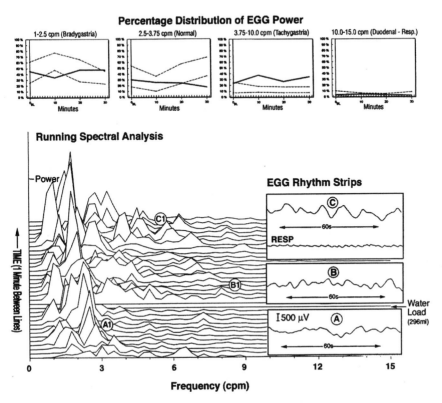

Figure 7.12. Tachygastria (diffuse pattern) with abnormal water load test. Electrogastrogram (EGG) rhythm strips, running spectral analysis (RSA), and percentage distribution of EGG power in a patient with chronic nausea. The EGG baseline rhythm strip (A) shows long-duration waves that are bradygastrias, but there are also low-amplitude faster frequencies in the EGG signal. The baseline RSA also shows a variety of peaks (A1). This patient ingested 296 ml of water during the water load, an abnormally low volume. The frequencies in the EGG rhythm strips vary from approximately 8 cpm in (B) to 5 cpm in (C). These frequencies are reflected in the RSA at (B1) and (C1). The percentage distribution of EGG power graphs show the bradygastria percentages are within the normal range or lower during the test, whereas the percentages in the normal range decrease throughout the post water load time period. In contrast, the tachygastria percentage increases at 10, 20, and 30 minutes after the water load. Thus, baseline EGG was within normal limits, but the water load evoked tachygastrias.

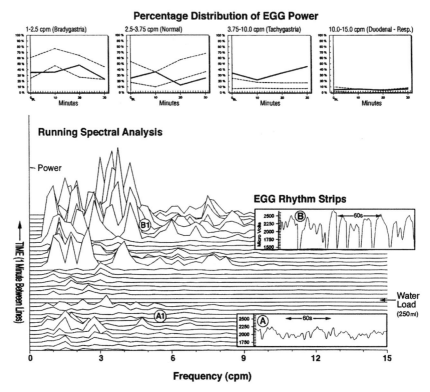

Figure 7.13. Tachygastria (diffuse pattern) with abnormal water load test. Electrogastrogram (EGG) rhythm strips, running spectral analysis (RSA), and percentage distribution of EGG power in a patient with chronic nausea. The EGG rhythm strip at baseline (A) shows a variety of frequencies. The patient ingested only 250 ml of water. The EGG rhythm strip B shows 4-cpm tachygastria. The baseline RSA shows peaks ranging from approximately 1, 3, and 5 cpm (A1). After ingestion of water there is little 3-cpm activity, a variety of peaks in the 1- to 2-cpm range, and then increased peaks around 4 and 8 cpm are seen toward the end of the RSA (B1). The percentage distribution of EGG power graphs show that the percentages in the bradygastria range are generally within normal limits. The percentage of normal 3-cpm power increases 10 minutes after ingestion of water but decreases below normal at 20 and 30 minutes. On the other hand, the percentage of EGG power in the tachygastria range increases 20 and 30 minutes after ingestion of water. Thus, overall the clinical diagnosis is a tachygastria and an abnormal water load test.

end of the recording. There also are other frequencies seen in the preceding minute of this EGG. The RSA from baseline shows peaks ranging from approximately 2 and 3 to 5 cpm.

After ingestion of water, there is little 3-cpm activity, and a variety of larger peaks in the 4- to 6- to 8-cpm tachygastria range are seen at (B1). The percentage distribution of EGG power shows that the percentages in the bradygastria range are within normal limits. The percentage of normal 3-cpm power increase 10 minutes after ingestion of water but decrease below normal at 20 and 30 minutes. The percentage of EGG power in the tachygastria at baseline range increased 20 and 30 minutes after the ingestion of water. In this example, the slight elevation in tachygastria present at baseline increased later after ingestion of the water load. The overall clinical diagnosis is a tachygastria and an abnormal water load test.

The water load test frequently evokes gastric dysrhythmias in patients who were in normal 3-cpm patterns during the baseline periods. An example of a diffuse tachygastria unmasked by the water load test is shown in Figure 7.14. In this case, very clear 3-cpm activity is present at baseline in the EGG rhythm strip (A) and in the RSA (A1). The series of tiny peaks at 6 and 9 cpm in the RSA at baseline are harmonics of the primary frequency (3 cpm). After ingestion of 237 ml of water, the EGG rhythm strip (B) shows a 6-cpm tachygastria. Corresponding peaks at 6 cpm are also seen in the RSA at (B1) after the ingestion of water. Thus, the peaks at (B1) in the RSA reflect the tachygastria seen in the EGG rhythm strip (B) and are not harmonics. Note also that after the water load there are no prominent 3-cpm peaks in the RSA. The percentage distribution of EGG power shows a high percentage of 3-cpm activity at baseline. After the ingestion of water, the percentage of EGG activity in the normal range decreases progressively. On the other hand, the percentage of power in the tachygastria range progressively increases 20 and 30 minutes after ingestion of water. In this case, ingestion of the water load evoked tachygastria. Thus, the clinical diagnosis is tachygastria (diffuse pattern) with an abnormal water load test.

This EGG may also be described by the prominent loss of 3-cpm activity after ingestion of the water load. This loss of 3-cpm activity, shown in Chapter 6 (Fig. 6.6), also has been described after ingestion of caloric meals.[38] In almost all cases, the loss of 3 cpm is replaced by a tachygastria as shown in Figure 7.14 or a flatline-type bradygastria.

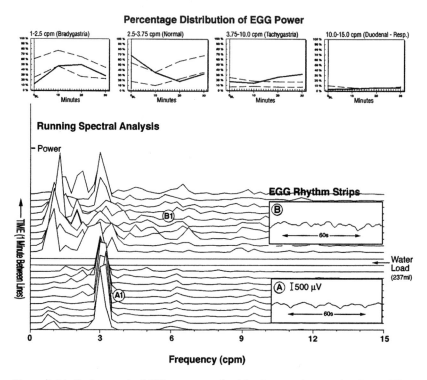

Figure 7.14. Tachygastria (diffuse pattern) with abnormal water load test. Electrogastrogram (EGG) rhythm strips, running spectral analysis (RSA), and percentage distribution of power from a patient with chronic nausea and vomiting. The baseline EGG shows a 3-cpm rhythm (A), and the baseline RSA shows 3-cpm peaks (A1). The series of tiny peaks at 6 and 9 cpm in the RSA at baseline are harmonics. After the ingestion of water, the EGG rhythm strip (B) shows an approximately 6-cpm tachygastria. Several small peaks at 6 cpm are also seen in the RSA at (B1). There are several peaks at 3 cpm and at 1 to 2 cpm as well. The percentage distribution of EGG power shows a high percentage of 3-cpm activity at baseline, but there is a progressive decrease in the normal EGG percentages after the water load. On the other hand, at 20 and 30 minutes after the ingestion of water, there is an increase in the percentage of EGG activity in the tachygastria range.

Tachygastrias (Probable)

Probable tachygastrias are diagnosed when several (1–5) minutes of EGG signal contain tachygastrias, but the EGG also contains many other minutes of normal 3-cpm activity.[8] These minutes of tachygastria activity are seen as peaks in the tachygastria range in the RSA and as increased percent distribution of power in the 3.75- to 10.0-cpm tachygastria range. However, these are probable tachygastrias because the percentage of 3-cpm activity remains in the normal ranges during the test period. Runs of tachygastria that occur briefly during the 30-minute post water load EGG recording can produce this pattern. In some patients, the raw EGG wave may carry two different frequencies: the normal 3-cpm waves and another frequency such as unifocal or diffuse tachygastria waves. In these patients, the normal pacemaker region apparently retains its rhythmicity, but an irritable focus generating the tachygastria is simultaneously active. (In recordings from dogs, the normal 5-cpm gastric pacesetter potential was recorded from the pacemaker region of the corpus, whereas 10-cpm tachygastrias were recorded simultaneously from the antrum.[36]) At other times, the 3-cpm activity disappears and is replaced for 1 or 2 minutes by a tachygastria (or bradygastria, as discussed later). In these instances, both 3-cpm activity and excessive tachygastria activity are present, and this pattern is termed *probable tachygastria.*

Figure 7.15 shows a probable tachygastria in a patient with unexplained nausea. The baseline EGG rhythm strip (A) shows a 4-cpm tachygastria. Respiration (RESP) is also shown. The RSA at (A1) also shows peaks at 4 cpm, which then evolve toward peaks at the normal 3-cpm frequency. During baseline, normal 3-cpm peaks were established just before the water load. The patient ingested 250 ml of water during the water load test. After the ingestion of water there was a brief increase in 6- to 7-cpm tachygastria (see EGG rhythm strip B) and the RSA at (B1). On the other hand, there also was some ongoing 3-cpm activity as shown by the 3-cpm peaks in the RSA after the water load. The percentage distribution of power shows that the EGG activity in the 3-cpm range was normal before and after the water load test but that tachygastria activity was increased at 20 and 30 minutes. Thus, the clinical EGG interpretation is "probable tachygastria" with an abnormal water load test.

Another example of a probable tachygastria in a patient with unexplained nausea is shown in Figure 7.16. The baseline EGG was

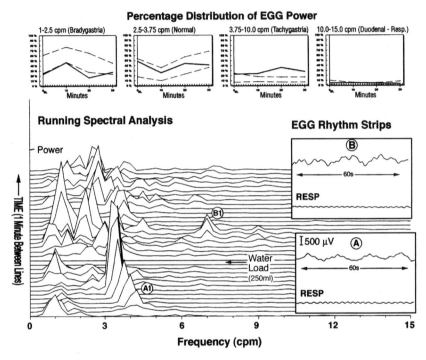

Percentage Distribution of EGG Power

1-2.5 cpm (Bradygastria)   2.5-3.75 cpm (Normal)   3.75-10.0 cpm (Tachygastria)   10.0-15.0 cpm (Duodenal - Resp.)

Running Spectral Analysis   **EGG Rhythm Strips**

Figure 7.15. Probable tachygastria with abnormal water load test. Electrogastrogram (EGG) rhythm strips, running spectral analysis (RSA), and percentage distribution of power from a patient with chronic nausea. The baseline EGG (A) shows a 4-cpm tachygastria. Respiration (RESP) is also shown. The RSA at (A1) also shows peaks at 4 cpm, which then evolve towards normal 3 cpm peaks. After the water load, a 6- to 7-cpm tachygastria developed briefly (see EGG rhythm strip B and the RSA at B1). On the other hand, 3-cpm activity continued as shown by the 3-cpm peaks in the RSA. The percentage distribution of power shows that the activity in the 3-cpm range was normal before and after the water load test. However, there was increased tachygastria activity 20 and 30 minutes after the water load test.

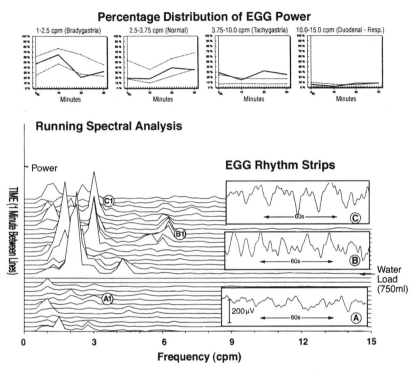

Percentage Distribution of EGG Power

1-2.5 cpm (Bradygastria)   2.5-3.75 cpm (Normal)   3.75-10.0 cpm (Tachygastria)   10.0-15.0 cpm (Duodenal - Resp.)

Figure 7.16. Probable tachygastria with normal water load test. Electrogastrogram (EGG) rhythm strips, running spectral analysis (RSA), and percentage distribution of EGG power before and after the water load test. The EGG rhythm strip at baseline (A) shows some 3-cpm activity. Similarly, the RSA at (A1) also shows a few peaks at 3 cpm. This patient ingested 750 ml as part of the water load test. After ingestion of the water load, increased 2-cpm peaks (the frequency dip) initially appear in the RSA. In the 20-minute period after the ingestion of water, however, the RSA shows a series of peaks in the 6-cpm range (B1). The EGG rhythm strip shown at B shows a 6-cpm tachygastria that lasted for several minutes. EGG rhythm strip (C) toward the end of the recording test shows return of 3-cpm EGG waves, and there are also peaks in the RSA at 3 cpm (C1) toward the end of the plot. The percentage distribution of EGG power shows a slight increase in tachygastria percentage at baseline, but tachygastria also increased at 20 minutes after the ingestion of water. The 3-cpm activity increased after ingestion of water at 10 and 20 minutes but decreased at minute 30. However, overall, the 3-cpm percentage activity was within the normal range. Thus, the overall EGG diagnosis is probable tachygastria with normal water load.

within normal limits and the patient ingested 750 ml of water during the water load test, a normal volume to ingest in the 5-minute period of time. Initially, there was the expected increase in 2-cpm activity (the frequency dip), but then several minutes of 6-cpm tachygastria developed, as seen in the EGG rhythm strip (B) and the RSA at (B1). Thereafter, however, the tachygastria disappeared and 3-cpm activity returned. The percentage distribution of EGG power mirrors this pattern and indicates an increase in the percentage of tachygastria activity at the 20-minute period after ingestion of water. Overall, however, a normal percentage of 3-cpm activity is also present. Therefore, this is a probable tachygastria.

It is interesting to note that in many of the tachygastrias, there is an increase in the percentage of tachygastria activity in the 10- and 20-minute periods after ingestion of the water volume. It is at this time that the stomach is maximally distended or stretched by the water volume, a physical stretch of the wall that may itself elicit transient gastric dysrhythmias in these patients. In patients with dyspepsia, nausea or bloating symptoms are generally increased during the 10 and 20 minutes after the water load is ingested.[17,32]

Fictitious Tachygastrias

Not all electrical waves that occur in the 3.7- to 10.0-cpm tachygastria range in the EGG rhythm strip or peaks that appear in the tachygastria range in the RSA (and thus not all percentages in the distribution of power in the tachygastria range) necessarily reflect tachygastrias. In some individuals, the respiratory rate is very slow and falls within the duodenal slow wave frequency or even tachygastria ranges. Electrical rhythms caused by diaphragmatic movement must be distinguished from gastric or duodenal myoelectrical rhythms. Figure 7.17 shows an EGG rhythm strip and RSA from a patient with recurrent nausea. The baseline RSA shows very few peaks at 3 cpm and a few 1- to 2-cpm peaks. After the ingestion of water, peaks appear in the RSA at 8 cpm (see the asterisk in Figure 7.17), and then peaks at 3 and 1 cpm increase in the last half of the RSA. Two minutes of the EGG signal and respiration signal recorded from the period immediately after ingestion of the water are shown in the inset. This patient was breathing at a very slow rate of approximately *8 breaths per minute* (see the asterisk in the inset in Fig. 7.17). The EGG rhythm is also approximately *8 cpm.* Thus, this is not a tachygastria but rather an 8-per-minute

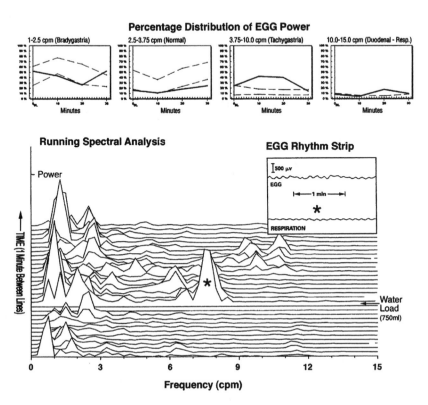

Figure 7.17. Fictitious tachygastria. Electrogastrogram (EGG) rhythm strips, running spectral analysis (RSA), and percentage distribution of power from a patient with chronic nausea and vomiting. The RSA at baseline shows very little 3-cpm peaks and several peaks in the 1- and 2-cpm range. After ingestion of water, peaks in the RSA at 8 cpm (*) are present. The EGG rhythm strip from that period of time (inset) shows a signal of approximately 8 cpm. Respiration recorded at the same time shows a respiratory rate of 8 breaths per minute. Therefore, the 8-cpm rhythm in the EGG is not a tachygastria but a respiratory rhythm. Toward the middle of the RSA, there are also peaks at 10 and 11 cpm that reflect an increase in respiration rate (respiration signal not shown). After the water load, some 3-cpm peaks appear in the RSA. The percentage distribution of power shows abnormally low percentages in the normal range. However, the increase in tachygastria activity at 10 and 20 minutes is likely due to the respiratory rhythms captured in the EGG and RSA. Thus, this is not a tachygastria; this is an abnormal EGG because there was a poor 3-cpm response to a normal volume of water.

respiratory rhythm reflected in the EGG recording. (Later in the recording, the respiratory rhythm increased to approximately 11 per minute as reflected by peaks at 11 cpm in the RSA.)

The percentage distribution of EGG power graphs in Figure 7.17 show abnormally low percentages of EGG power in the normal range after the water load. However, the increase in the percentages of tachygastria power at 10 and 20 minutes is due to the respiratory signals. Thus, this is an abnormal EGG because there was a very poor 3-cpm response to a normal volume of water. The clinical interpretation is not a tachygastria, because the tachygastria peaks in the RSA and the percentage of tachygastria power were caused by the respiratory signals.

Figure 7.18 shows another example of fictitious tachygastria. The baseline RSA shows 3-cpm peaks and varying peaks from 7 to 9 cpm. Thus, both normal 3-cpm frequencies and tachygastria frequencies were present at baseline. A normal water volume (700 ml) was ingested. Many RSA peaks at 3 cpm (A1) were elicited after the water load. At the same time, there are peaks at 6 cpm in the RSA after the water load. Review of the EGG rhythm strip (A) after the water load shows 3-cpm EGG waves are present. This patient's respiration (RESP) rate was approximately 6 per minute, however, and small 6-per-minute waves that reflect the respiratory rate are carried in the 3-cpm EGG signal. Thus, the 6-cpm peaks in the RSA represent the 6-per-minute respiration rate. The percentage distribution of EGG power shows that there is a normal distribution of power in the normal range until minute 30 after the water load. The percentage of EGG power in the tachygastria range reflects the very slow 6-per-minute respiratory rate in this patient. Thus, the clinical interpretation of this EGG is a normal EGG with normal water load test.

Peaks in the tachygastria range in the RSA may also reflect harmonics (see Chapter 4 and Fig. 4.6). However, in the case of harmonics, a clear primary frequency (e.g., 3 cpm) is also present in the RSA. The strong peaks at 3 cpm in the RSA are accompanied by a parallel set of low-power peaks at 6 and even lower-power peaks at 9 cpm to form the obvious "harmonics" of the primary frequency. Furthermore, if frequency peaks in the tachygastria range in the RSA represent harmonics, then inspection of the raw EGG signal reveals *no* 6- or 9-cpm EGG waves (see Figs. 7.4 and 7.14 at baseline), but clear 3-cpm EGG waves will be present. (The presence of harmonics in the RSA analyses or brief intermittent tachygastrias in healthy

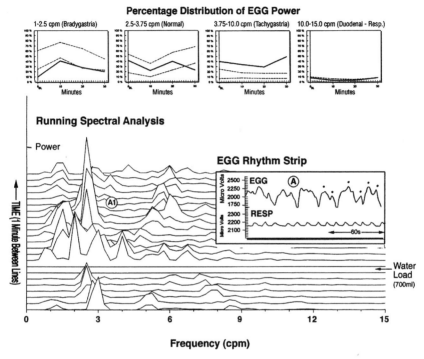

Figure 7.18. Fictitious tachygastria. Electrogastrogram (EGG) rhythm strips, running spectral analysis (RSA), and percentage distribution of power from a patient with persistent nausea. The baseline RSA shows 3 cpm peaks. Peaks are also seen at 7 to 9 cpm. A normal water volume (700 ml) was ingested. After the water load, many peaks at 3 cpm in the RSA (A1) were elicited. Peaks at 6 cpm in the RSA also developed after the water load. Review of the EGG rhythm strip (A) after the water load shows 3-cpm EGG waves are present, but at the same time this patient's respiration (RESP) rate was approximately 6 per minute. There are small 6-per-minute waves in the 3-cpm EGG signal that reflect this respiratory rate (black dots). Thus, the 6-cpm peaks in the RSA represent the 6-per-minute respiration rate. The percentage distribution of EGG power shows that there is a normal distribution of power in the normal range until minute 30. The persistent tachygastria percentages reflect the slow 6-per-minute respiratory rate in this patient. This is a normal EGG with normal water load test.

subjects accounts for the 20% or less of all of the EGG power in the tachygastria range that is displayed in the percentage distribution graphs.[17])

Summary

The spectrum of tachygastrias presented in the chapter show the many patterns of abnormally fast gastric dysrhythmias recorded with EGG methods in patients with unexplained nausea, vomiting, and dyspepsia symptoms. Tachygastrias correlate with nausea symptoms and are associated with more delayed gastric emptying compared with bradygastria. Pitfalls in the EGG analysis include misidentifying harmonics or respiratory rhythms as tachygastrias. These pitfalls can be easily avoided by careful inspection of the raw EGG signal and the respiratory rhythm. An approach to treatment of patients with gastric dysrhythmias and tachygastrias was outlined in Chapter 6. Future investigations of the basic mechanisms of tachygastrias will lead to innovative approaches to therapies of these dysrhythmias.

References

1. Koch KL: Electrogastrography. In: Schuster M, Crowell M, Koch KL, eds. *Atlas of Gastrointestinal Motility*. Hamilton, Ontario, Canada: BC Decker; 2002.
2. Hinder RA, Kelley KA: Human gastric pacesetter potential: site of origin, spread, and response to gastric transection and proximal vagotomy. *Am J Surg* 1997;133:29–33.
3. Smout AJPM, van der Schee EJ, Grashuis JL: What is measured in electrogastrography? *Dig Dis Sci* 1980;25:179–187.
4. You CH, Chey WY, Lee KY, et al: Gastric and small intestinal myoelectric dysrhythmia associated with chronic intractable nausea and vomiting. *Ann Intern Med* 1981;95:449–451.
5. Familoni BO, Bowes KL, Kingma WJ, et al: Can transcutaneous recordings detect gastric electrical abnormalities? *Gut* 1991;32:141–146.
6. Koch KL, Stern RM, Vasey M, et al: Gastric dysrhythmias and nausea of pregnancy. *Dig Dis Sci* 1990;35:961–968.
7. Amaris MA, Sanmiguel CP, Sadowski DC, et al: Electrical activity from colon overlaps with normal gastric electrical activity in cutaneous recordings. *Dig Dis Sci* 2002;47:2480–2485.
8. Verhagan MAMT, van Schelven AJ, Samsom M, et al: Pitfalls of the analysis of electrogastrographic recordings. *Gastroenterology* 1999;117:453–460.

9. Abell TL, Malagelada J-R. Glucagon-evoked gastric dysrhythmias in humans shown by an improved electrogastrographic technique. *Gastroenterology* 1985; 88:1932–1940.

10. Stern RM, Leibowitz HW, Unblad I, et al: Tachygastria and motion sickness. *Aviat Space Environ Med* 1985;56:1074–1077.

11. Geldof H, van der Schee EJ, van Blankenstein M, et al: Electrogastrographic study of gastric myoelectrical activity in patients with unexplained nausea and vomiting. *Gut* 1986;27:799–808.

12. Chen J, Schirmer BD, McCallum RW: Serosal and cutaneous recordings of gastric myoelectrical activity in patients with gastroparesis. *Am J Physiol* 1994; 206:G90–G98.

13. Chaap HM, Smout AJPM, Akkermans LM: Myoelectric activity of the Bilroth II gastric remnant. *Gut* 1990;31:984–988.

14. Thunberg L: Interstitial cells of Cajal. In: Wood JD, ed. *The Handbook of Physiology, The Gastrointestinal System, Section 6, Vol 1, Part 1.* Bethesda, MD:1989:349–386.

15. Huisinga JD: Physiology and pathophysiology of the interstitial cell of Cajal: from bench to bedside, II. Gastric motility: lessons from mutant mice on slow waves and innervation. *Am J Physiol* 2001;281:G1129–G1134.

16. Kim TW, Beckett EAH, Hanna R, et al: Regulation of pacemaker frequency in the murine gastric antrum. *J Physiol* (Lond) 2002;538:145–157.

17. Koch KL, Hong S-P, Xu L: Reproducibility of gastric myoelectrical activity and the water load test in patients with dysmotility-like dyspepsia symptoms and in control subjects. *J Clin Gastroenterol* 2000;31:125–129.

18. Jebbink HJA, Bruijs PPM, Varvenboer B, et al: Gastric myoelectrical activity in patients with type I diabetes mellitus and autonomic neuropathy. *Dig Dis Sci* 1994;39:2376–2383.

19. Schreibman I, Xu L, Carusone S, et al: Water load test unmasks nausea, bloating and tachygastria in patients with type 2 diabetes mellitus. *Neurogastroenterol Motil* 2001;13:274.

20. Hasler WL, Soudah HC, Dulai G, et al: Mediation of hyperglycemia-evoked gastric slow wave dysrhythmias by endogenous prostaglandins. *Gastroenterology* 1995;108:727–736.

21. Sarna S: In vivo myoelectrical activity: methods, analysis and interpretation. In: Schultz S, Wood JD, eds. *Handbook of Physiology: The Gastrointestinal System.* Baltimore, MD: Waverly Press; 1989:817–863.

22. Stoddard CJ, Smallwood RH, Duthie HL: Electrical arrhythmias in the human stomach. *Gut* 1981;22:705–712.

23. Kim CG, Hanson RB, Abell TL, et al: Effect of inhibition of prostaglandin synthesis on epinephrine-induced gastroduodenal electromechanical changes in humans. *Mayo Clin Proc* 1989;64:149–157.

24. Xu L, Koch KL, Summy-Long J, et al: Hypothalamic and gastric myoelectrical responses during vection-induced nausea in healthy Chinese subject. *Am J Physiol* 1993;265:E578–E584.

25. Uitjtdehaage SHJ, Stern RM, Koch KL: Effects of eating on vection-induced motion sickness, cardiac vagal tone and gastric myoelectrical activity. *Psychophysiology* 1992;29:193–201.

26. Koch KL, Stern RM: Functional disorders of the stomach. *Semin Gastroenterol* 1990;1:23–36.

27. Kohagen KR, Kim MS, McDonnell WM, et al: Nicotine effects of prostaglandin-dependent gastric slow wave rhythmicity and antral motility in non-smokers and smokers. *Gastroenterology* 1996;110:3–11.

28. Walsh JW, Hasler WL, Nugent CE, et al: Progesterone and estrogen are potential mediators of gastric slow wave dysrhythmias in nausea of pregnancy. *Am J Physiol* 1996;270:G506–G514.

29. Ordog T, Baldo M, Danko R, et al: Plasticity of electrical pacemaking by interstitial cells of Cajal and gastric dysrhythmias in W/W^v mutant mice. *Gastroenterology* 2002;123:2028–2040.

30. Koch KL, Dwyer A, Jeffries GH: Electromechanical effects of indomethacin on in vivo rabbit ileum. *Am J Physiol* 1986;250:G135–G139.

31. Devane SP, Ravelli AM, Bisset WM, et al: Gastric antral dysrhythmias in children with chronic idiopathic intestinal pseudoobstruction. *Gut* 1992;33:1477–1481.

32. Boeckxstaens GE, Hirsch DP, van den Elzen BDJ, et al: Impaired drinking capacity in patients with functional dyspepsia: relationship with proximal stomach function. *Gastroenterology* 2001;121:1054–1064.

33. Gilija OH, Hausken T, Wilhelmsen I, et al: Impaired accomodation of proximal stomach to a meal in functional dyspepsia. *Dig Dis Sci* 1996;41:689–696.

34. Gilija OH, Detmer PR, Jong JM, et al: Intragastric distribution and gastric emptying assessed by three-dimensional ultrasonography. *Gastroenterology* 1997;113:38–49.

35. Noar M, Koch KL, Xu L: Spectrum of gastric neuromuscular dysfunction in patients with GERD and dysmotility-like functional dyspepsia (GERD+). *Am J Gastroenterol* 2002;122:416A.

36. Code CF, Marlett JA: Canine tachygastria. *Mayo Clin Proc* 1974;49:325–332.

37. Mintchev M, Otto SJ, Bowes KL: Electrogastrography can recognize gastric electrical uncoupling in dogs. *Gastroenterology* 1997;112:2006–2011.

38. Lin Z, Chen JDZ, Schirmer BD, et al: Postprandial response of gastric slow waves: correlation of serosal recordings with the electrogastrogram. *Dig Dis Sci* 2000;45:645–651.

8

Bradygastrias and Mixed Dysrhythmias

*B*radygastrias are low-frequency electrogastrogram (EGG) waves that range from approximately 1.0 to 2.5 cycles per minute (cpm).[1-8] Some bradygastria waves are high amplitude and occupy the full scale of the EGG recording channel; others are very low amplitude and appear to be almost flatline. Bradygastrias have been recorded in patients with functional dyspepsia,[9,10] diabetic and idiopathic gastropathy,[11,12] and nausea of pregnancy.[13] These patients have symptoms of abdominal discomfort, fullness, nausea, and vomiting. In this chapter, the causes of bradygastria patterns are reviewed and examples of bradygastrias are shown. EGGs also may have increased bradygastria *and* tachygastria waves, a pattern termed a *mixed dysrhythmia.*

Origin of Bradygastrias

Slow-Frequency Contractions of Antrum and Fundus

The exact origin of bradygastrias has been difficult to determine. In certain circumstances, the antrum contracts at 1.5 to 1.8 contractions per minute rather than the more recognized 3-per-minute contractions.[14] Figure 8.1 indicates the relationship between EGG waves and low-frequency antral peristaltic contractions recorded from an intraluminal pressure sensing device during fasting and after infusion of erythromycin in healthy individuals.[14] The antral contractions were recorded 3 and 1.5 cm from the pylorus. During fasting, 2-cpm EGG waves were present and correlated with 2-per-minute antral contractions. Each of these low-frequency contractions was associated with a low-frequency EGG wave (a negative deflection followed by a positive deflection). Irregular antral attractions also occur during fasting and may be reflected in the EGG as 1- to 2-cpm EGG waves. After erythromycin infusion, the EGG waves occurred at 1.0 to 1.5 cpm and correlated with stronger antral contractions that occurred at the same frequency: 1.0 to 1.5 per minute. Thus, the bradygastria EGG frequencies correlated with the low-frequency antral contractions during fasting and after infusion of erythromycin. These studies indicate that, under certain conditions, bradygastria waves reflect low-frequency antral contractions.

The fundus of the stomach normally contracts slowly at a rate from 0.5 to 1 contraction per minute.[15] Thus, the low-frequency contractile activity of the fundus may also be reflected in the low-frequency EGG signals in certain situations.

Temperature of Intragastric Content

Bradygastrias may be transiently recorded in healthy individuals, especially during fasting. In the first 10 minutes after the water load test, a "frequency dip" occurs during which the frequency of the EGG decreases transiently into the 2.0- to 2.5-cpm range (see Chapter 3). The frequency dip is transient, however, and in the 20- and 30-minute periods after ingestion of the water, normal 3-cpm EGG waves develops in healthy individuals. Why does the frequency dip occur? Smout et al.[3] showed that decreasing the temperature of ingested water alters the frequency dip that is seen initially after ingestion of water, yogurt, and a variety of other foods. When body temperature water (37°C) was ingested, the frequency dip was *not* induced and the normal 3-cpm EGG activity was initiated immediately after the water load. On the other hand, ingestion of 4°C water induced the frequency dip with the normal EGG rhythm decreasing into the bradygastria range[16] (Fig. 8.2). These studies indicate that

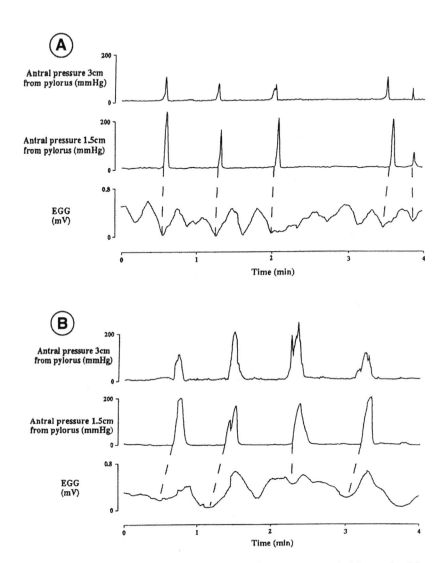

Figure 8.1. Electrogastrogram (EGG) and antral pressure recorded from a healthy subject during fasting and after erythromycin infusion. (*A*) During fasting, 2-cpm EGG waves are associated with phase II antral contractions (*B*). After erythromycin infusion, 1- to 2-cpm EGG waves are associated with high-amplitude 1-2-per-minute antral contractions. (From Sun et al., with permission.)

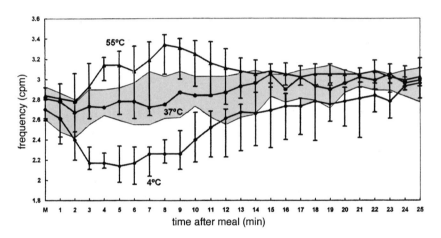

Figure 8.2. EGG recordings from healthy subjects after ingestion of cold (4°C) and warm (37°C) water. Note the decrease in EGG wave frequency after ingestion of the cold water compared with the body temperature water. (From Verhagon et al., with permission.)

the temperature of the ingested material has an effect on gastric myoelectrical rhythmicity. Thus, ingestion of several hundred milliliters of cool water is one factor that slows the EGG frequency associated with the frequency dip.

Intragastric Volume

There are other factors that induce low-frequency gastric pacesetter potential activity and lower the EGG frequency. Lin et al.[17] showed that the volume of water instilled into the canine stomach was inversely related to gastric pacesetter potential frequency (Fig. 8.3). The normal 4.5-cpm canine pacesetter potential frequency decreased to 2.5 cpm as the volume of body temperature water infused into the stomach over a 5-minute period was increased from 150 to 1800 ml. The pacesetter potential frequency gradually returned to the baseline 5 cpm during the subsequent 30-minute period. Tachygastrias did not occur during or after gastric distention with water in the healthy dogs. The temporary decrease in slow wave frequency after the infusion of water volumes in dogs is analogous to the transient frequency dips into the bradygastria range that is seen during the EGG response to the water load test in healthy subjects[4] (see Figs. 3.13, 3.14, and 3.15).

Distention of Antrum

Figure 8.4 shows that bradygastrias also are induced by distention of the antrum. In these studies in healthy subjects, a barostat balloon was used to distend the antrum and then the fundus.[18] During the basal condition with no balloon distention, 3-cpm EGG signals were recorded. During balloon distention of the antrum, healthy subjects developed nausea and bradygastria. Distention of the fundus evoked neither dysrhythmias nor nausea. In patients with unexplained nausea and dysmotility-like dyspepsia, distention or stretch of the corpus antrum with water loading evokes bradygastrias (and tachygastrias) and nausea. Thus, the bradygastrias evoked by gastric distention with noncaloric meals most likely originate from the antrum.

Figure 8.5 shows an EGG recorded from a patient who had a very clear 2-cpm EGG pattern in the first 15 minutes after the water load test. The 2-cpm EGG waves are clearly seen in the EGG rhythm strip and are reminiscent of the slow-frequency EGG signals after

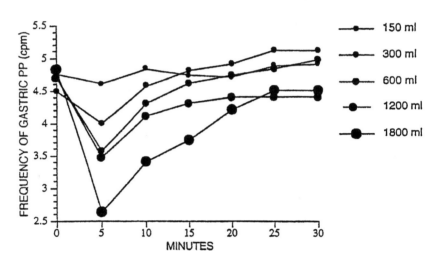

Figure 8.3. Volume of buffered water solution in stomach versus canine gastric slow wave frequency. With increasing volume in the stomach, gastric slow wave frequency transiently decreases. (From Lin et al., with permission.)

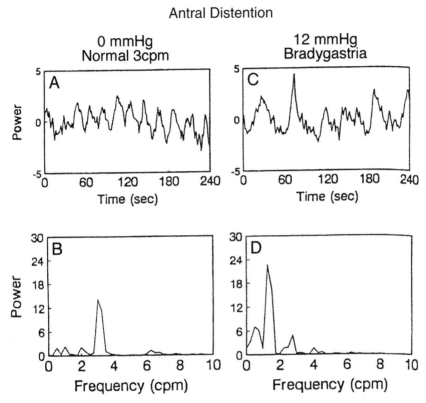

Figure 8.4. The effects of antral distention on electrogastrogram (EGG) activity in healthy individuals. Distention was accomplished by inflating a barostat balloon in the antrum. The panels labeled Basal indicates 0 mmHg pressure in the bag. The top panel shows normal 3-cpm EGG (*A*) activity, and the Fourier transform of the EGG signal below (*B*) shows a peak at 3 cpm. On the other hand, when the balloon was distended to 12 mmHg, a bradygastria pattern was recorded as shown in the EGG with 1- to 2-cpm waves (*C*), and the Fourier transform of the EGG signal shows increased power at 1 to 1.5 cpm (*D*). (Modified from San Miguel et al., with permission.)

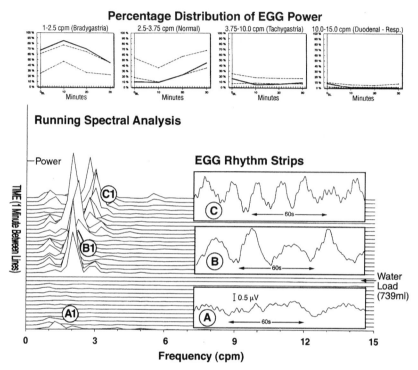

Percentage Distribution of EGG Power

1-2.5 cpm (Bradygastria) 2.5-3.75 cpm (Normal) 3.75-10.0 cpm (Tachygastria) 10.0-15.0 cpm (Duodenal - Resp.)

Minutes   Minutes   Minutes   Minutes

Running Spectral Analysis

Power

TIME (1 Minute Between Lines)

EGG Rhythm Strips

C1

B1

A1

C

B

A

60s

60s

60s

I 0.5 μV

Water
Load
(739ml)

0   3   6   9   12   15

Frequency (cpm)

Figure 8.5. Bradygastria after a normal water load. Electrogastrogram (EGG) rhythm strips, running spectral analysis (RSA), and percentage distribution of EGG power in a patient with unexplained nausea. Baseline EGG rhythm strips (A) show some 1- to 2-cpm waves. After ingestion of a 739 ml water load, large-amplitude 2-cpm EGG waves are seen (B). By 30 minutes after the water load, the EGG rhythm strip shows 3-cpm waves (C). The RSA at baseline (A1) is very flat due to scaling needed to plot the high-power peaks after the water load. After ingestion of water, 2-cpm peaks in the RSA are seen at (B1) and peaks at 3 cpm appear later (C1) in the RSA. The bradygastria percentages are above normal throughout this test, 3-cpm activity is below normal until the 30 minutes after water ingestion. Percentages of total EGG power in the tachygastria and duodenal range are normal. Overall, this is a brachygastria and normal water load test.

192

erythromycin (see Fig. 8.1). In the last part of this recording, however, normal 3-cpm EGG waves developed. Thus, this was a bradygastria and normal water load test, with an early pronounced low-frequency dip.

Transection of the Gastric Corpus and Bradygastria

San Miguel et al.[19] incised circumferentially the canine corpus and antrum and recorded pacesetter potential activity from serosal electrodes. In the antrum, the pacesetter potential frequency decreased from 5 cpm before the incision to 1 to 2 cpm after the incision. Thus, it is clear that the incised antrum, dissected from the normal pacesetter potential region, has an intrinsic low-frequency rhythm in the bradygastria range. Similarly, antral slow wave frequency decreased from 3.5 to 1.5 cpm in the murine antrum after circumferential incision of the corpus.[20] Thus, bradygastria may also originate from the antrum under certain experimental postsurgical conditions as the intrinsic slow pacesetter potential frequency of the antrum is unmasked by surgical uncoupling the antrum from the corpus.[19,20]

Colonic and Small Intestinal Myoelectrical Activity

Nongastric myoelectrical activity may be recorded with the EGG electrodes as described in this text. The colon contracts at irregular times and occasionally at low frequencies from 1 to 3 per minute. Thus, some low-frequency components in the EGG, especially during fasting when the stomach electrical rhythm is relatively unstable, may reflect colonic myoelectrical events. Colectomy reduces these low-frequency components in the EGG signal.[21,22] The gastrocolonic reflex is stimulated after caloric meals, and postprandial colonic contractions may be reflected in the EGG signal. Thus, caloric meals may elicit undesirable colonic contractions that contaminate the EGG signal in the postprandial period. On the other hand, phase III antral and small bowel contractions occur during fasting and may affect the EGG signal, as discussed in Chapter 3. The water load test contributes to reliable EGG recordings because it provides a standard pretest snack and a noncaloric challenge for stomach neuromuscular activity without calorie-induced hormonal or other neurohormonal effects that stimulate colonic electrocontractile activity.[23]

Movements of the Body and Limbs of the Subject

One of the most common causes of low-frequency waves in the EGG is a deep breath or cough. Such events are often associated with movement of the abdomen that creates an obvious high-amplitude artifact wave in the EGG signal. Movement of the limbs may also cause low-frequency and high-amplitude waves.[8] By recording respiration concomitantly with the EGG signal, these events can be detected and eliminated from visual and computer analysis.

To summarize, the origin of bradygastrias is likely the antrum since 1- to 2.5-cpm pacesetter potential frequencies are the intrinsic antral frequencies. However, the volume and temperature of ingested liquids slow EGG frequency temporarily, and distention of the antrum also induces bradygastria. Clinicians and investigators need to be cognizant of these variables when recording EGGs.

Taken together, the many studies of EGG rhythms indicate that the normal human gastric pacesetter potential rhythm is not fixed at 3 cpm. There is considerable plasticity and flexibility in the repertoire of normal gastric myoelectrical rhythms.[1,8,9] The ongoing gastric myoelectrical frequency reflects the ongoing fasting, postprandial, or environmental circumstances. For example, healthy individuals develop EGG frequencies in the bradygastria range transiently after the water load test, the "frequency dip." The normal 3-cpm EGG activity is reestablished after the initial myoelectrical response to the volume and temperature attributes of the water load. On the other hand, patients with nausea and unexplained dyspepsia symptoms have relatively fixed bradygastrias or develop sustained bradygastrias after the water load test.

Bradygastrias

In the next section, bradygastrias that were recorded from patients are presented. These examples illustrate the variety of bradygastria EGG patterns that are elicited by the water load test.

Bradygastria (High Amplitude)

A high-amplitude bradygastria after a water load of 739 ml is shown in Figure 8.5. The clear 2-cpm bradygastria occurs in the first 10 minutes after ingestion of water and is considered the normal frequency

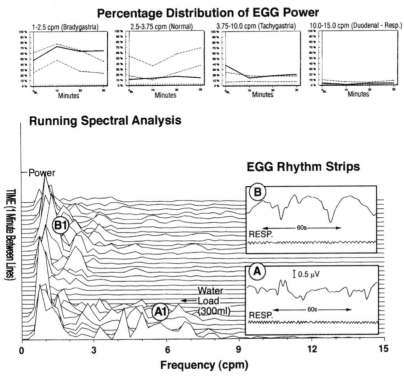

Percentage Distribution of EGG Power

1-2.5 cpm (Bradygastria) 2.5-3.75 cpm (Normal) 3.75-10.0 cpm (Tachygastria) 10.0-15.0 cpm (Duodenal - Resp.)

Minutes Minutes Minutes Minutes

Running Spectral Analysis

Power

TIME (1 Minute Between Lines)

B1

EGG Rhythm Strips

B

RESP. ← 60s →

A

I 0.5 µV

Water
←Load→
(300ml)

RESP. ← 60s →

A1

Frequency (cpm)

0   3   6   9   12   15

Figure 8.6. Bradygastria after a abnormal water load. Electrogastrogram (EGG) rhythm strips, running spectral analysis (RSA), and percentage distribution of EGG power from a patient with functional dyspepsia are shown. The baseline EGG rhythm strip (A) shows a variety of frequencies in the signal. In the baseline RSA a variety of peaks are seen (A1). After ingestion of a low volume of water (300 ml), 1- to 2-cpm bradygastria waves increased as shown in the EGG rhythm strip (B). The increased 1- to 2-cpm waves are mirrored in the increased peaks in the 1- to 2-cpm range in the RSA (B1). After ingestion of the water the increased percentage of tachygastria activity at baseline disappeared and bradygastria activity increased to the upper limits of normal and then into the abnormal range by 30 minutes.

dip described in Chapter 3. This figure shows the EGG rhythm strips, running spectral analysis (RSA), and percentage distribution of EGG power in a patient with unexplained nausea. Baseline EGG rhythm strip (A) show some 1- to 2-cpm waves. After ingestion of the water load, large-amplitude 2-cpm EGG waves are seen (B). By 30 minutes after the water load, the EGG rhythm strip shows clear 3-cpm waves (C). The RSA at baseline (A1) is very flat because of the scaling needed to graph the high-power waves after the water load. After the ingestion of water, 2-cpm peaks in the RSA are seen (B1). These peaks correspond with the 2-cpm EGG waves seen in the EGG rhythm strip (B). Later in the RSA, the peaks at 3 cpm appear (C1) and correspond to the 3-cpm EGG waves in the rhythm strip (C). The percentage distribution of EGG power indicates that the normal 3-cpm activity is below normal until the 30-minute period after water ingestion. Percentages of tachygastrias and duodenal activity are normal, but the bradygastria percentages are above normal throughout this test. Thus, the clinical diagnosis is bradygastria and normal water load test.

The baseline EGG recording is made during fasting and the rhythm may be unstable. The water load test stimulates the gastric neuromuscular apparatus to respond to volume and distention. A normal 3-cpm EGG pattern may develop or a gastric neuromuscular dysrhythmia may develop. Figure 8.6 shows a high-amplitude bradygastria dysrhythmia recorded from a 25-year-old patient with unexplained nausea. In this recording, the baseline EGG rhythm strip (A) shows a variety of frequencies, that is, an unstable fasting EGG rhythm. In the RSA from the baseline recording, a variety of peaks at 1 to 2 cpm and 5 and 7 cpm are seen (A1). The patient ingested a low volume of water (300 ml). After the ingestion of water, there was increased 1- to 2-cpm activity as shown in the EGG rhythm strip (B). The increased 1- to 2-cpm EGG waves are mirrored in the RSA with increased peaks at 1 to 2 cpm (B1). The percentage distribution of EGG power showed increased tachygastria at baseline, but after the ingestion of water, the tachygastria disappeared, and bradygastria activity increased to the upper limits of normal and then into the abnormal range by the 30-minute period. The overall diagnosis is bradygastria with abnormal water load.

In other patients, a baseline bradygastria is present and may reflect stomach or colonic myoelectrical activity, but the water load evokes clear 1- to 2-cpm waves and indicates bradygastria. In Figure 8.7, for example, low-amplitude 1- to 2-cpm EGG signals are present in the baseline rhythm strip (A), but high-amplitude 1- to 2-cpm EGG

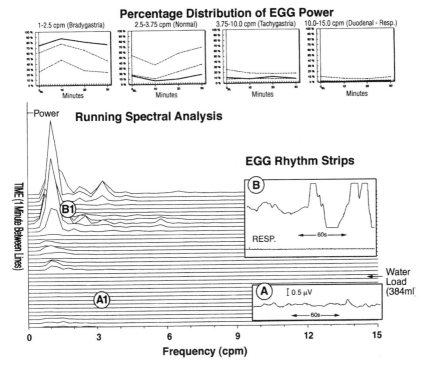

Figure 8.7. Bradygastria with abnormal water load test. Electrogastrogram (EGG) rhythm strips, running spectral analysis (RSA), and percentage distribution of EGG power in a patient with dysmotility-like dyspepsia symptoms are shown. The baseline EGG rhythm strip showed a low amplitude irregular signal (A). The patient ingested 384 ml of water during the water load test and in the 20- to 30-minute time period after the ingestion of water several large-amplitude 1-cpm waves were recorded (B). The RSA shows the high-power 1-cpm peaks after ingestion of water at (B1). Several small peaks at 3 cpm are also seen. The peaks at 1 cpm are scaled according to the power of frequencies in the EGG. Therefore, the RSA lines during baseline are flat because power of EGG frequencies was very small compared with power after the water load (B1). The percentage distribution of EGG power show a very poor 3-cpm activity throughout the recording and persistent increases in the bradygastria activity.

197

waves occurred about 25 minutes after the water load, as shown in the EGG rhythm strip (B). Respiration rate had not changed, and body movements that might have created the 1- to 2-cpm EGG were not noted. Thus, the high-amplitude 1- to 2-cpm EGG waves most likely reflected gastric contractions. The high-amplitude EGG signal waves are represented in the RSA as the high-power 1- to 2-cpm peaks shown (B1). Baseline peaks in the RSA are suppressed due to scaling needed to plot the high-power 1- to 2-cpm peaks after the water load. The high-amplitude 1- to 2-cpm EGG waves and 1- to 2-cpm peaks in the RSA are also are reflected in the increased percentage of EGG power in the 1- to 2-cpm range, especially at 20 and 30 minutes after the water load. This EGG is interpreted as a bradygastria with decreased water load volume.

Bradygastria (Low Amplitude)

A normal baseline 3-cpm rhythm may be markedly disrupted in some patients after distention of the stomach with the physical volume of water or a caloric meal. In the EGG and water load test from a patient with recurrent nausea shown in Figure 8.8, the baseline rhythm strip (A) shows a normal 3-cpm pattern. The patient ingested 450 ml of water. Under the conditions of loading (stretching) the stomach with the water load, the normal 3-cpm rhythm response *did not* develop and a low-amplitude bradygastria was elicited as shown (B). The RSA of the baseline EGG signal shows regular peaks at 3 cpm (A1). After the ingestion of a near-normal volume of water (450 ml), the 3-cpm peaks disappear, several high-power 1- to 2-cpm peaks are seen, and only low-power 1- to 2-cpm peaks are noted for the remainder of the study. This marked loss of normal 3-cpm activity after a meal may be considered a separate diagnostic pattern (as described in Chapter 6, see Fig. 6.6) or a low-amplitude bradygastria. The percentage distribution of EGG power graphs show this pattern very clearly. At baseline, almost 55% of the EGG power was in the normal range. The percentage in the normal range fell dramatically after the water load, whereas the bradygastria percentage of EGG power increased above the normal range. Thus, this is a bradygastria.

After the provocative water load test, the 3-cpm rhythm may disappear as shown earlier, or unstable baseline rhythms develop into clear bradygastria rhythms. In these patients, the stretch of the neuromuscular wall of the stomach by the water load elicits the gastric

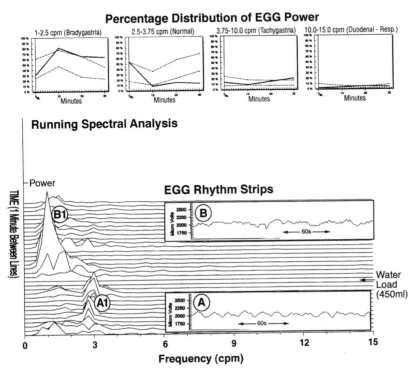

Percentage Distribution of EGG Power

1-2.5 cpm (Bradygastria) 2.5-3.75 cpm (Normal) 3.75-10.0 cpm (Tachygastria) 10.0-15.0 cpm (Duodenal - Resp.)

Running Spectral Analysis

EGG Rhythm Strips

Figure 8.8. Bradygastria with abnormal water load test. Electrogastrogram (EGG) rhythm strips, running spectral analysis (RSA), and percentage distribution of EGG power are shown from a patient with bloating and nausea. The baseline EGG rhythm strip shows a consistent 3 cpm signal (A) and regular peaks at 3 cpm are seen in the baseline periods of the RSA (A1). After ingestion of the water load, there was virtually no 3-cpm EGG response (B) and no 3-cpm peaks in the RSA. The peaks in the RSA are in the 1- to 2-cpm range (B1). The percentage distribution of EGG power in the 3-cpm range is normal at baseline. After ingestion of water, the percentage 3-cpm activity abruptly decreased to below normal levels while the percentage of power in the bradygastria range increased above normal levels.

neuromuscular response of the sustained 1- to 2-cpm EGG rhythms. The bradygastria patterns shown here most likely reflect abnormal antral myoelectrical activity evoked by the water load, because movement artifact is identified and eliminated, water temperature is controlled, and fundic or colonic contractions are unlikely.

Mixed Gastric Dysrhythmias

Mixed gastric dysrhythmias are diagnosed when the EGG signals contain bradygastria *and* tachygastria waves after the water load test. Normal 3-cpm EGG activity may also occur transiently during mixed dysrhythmias. Thus, this myoelectrical response to the ingestion of water is diagnosed as a mixed or nonspecific gastric dysrhythmia. These rhythms may be difficult to diagnose from the raw EGG signals because of the varying pattern of frequencies in the EGG signal after the water load test. The origins of mixed dysrhythmias are unknown but likely are caused by elements described for bradygastria in this chapter and for tachygastrias in Chapter 7.

In patients with functional dysmotility-like dyspepsia and in a cohort of patients with type 2 diabetes mellitus, mixed gastric dysrhythmias were uncommon.[4,9] However, patients with gastroesophageal reflux disease and dysmotility-like dyspepsia (GERD+) had a high percentage of mixed dysrhythmias that were unmasked by the water load test.[23] Forty percent of these patients had gastric dysrhythmias at baseline, but 79% had gastric dysrhythmias after the water load test.[24] These findings raise the possibility that the mixed dysrhythmia is a specific dysrhythmia associated with GERD and dyspepsia symptoms. When the lower esophageal sphincter relaxes inappropriately during the gastric neuromuscular work of emptying the water load, then a transient loss of intragastric pressure occurs, an event that may affect ongoing gastric neuromuscular activity and stimulate a mixed gastric dysrhythmia. Studies are needed to further define the relationships among mixed dysrhythmias, transient lower esophageal sphincter relaxations, and GERD.

Abnormalities in the function of interstitial cells, smooth muscle cells, enteric neurons, or alterations in paracrine or hormone response systems also may underlie mixed dysrhythmias. Tachygastrias usually develop initially after the water load and suggest that the distention or stretch of the antrum or corpus elicits the dysrhythmia.

The bradygastrias develop during the 20 to 30 minutes after the water load, suggesting fundic and/or antral contractions develop in an atypical fashion in the patients with GERD+. Various examples of mixed dysrhythmias are presented next.

A mixed dysrhythmia in a patient with dysmotility-like dyspepsia symptoms is shown in Figure 8.9. The EGG rhythm strip from baseline contains signals from 1 to 2 cpm (A). The RSA of the baseline EGG signal shows large peaks at 1 to 2 cpm (A1). The patient ingested 400 ml of water during the water load test. The EGG rhythm strip (B) shows normal 3-cpm waves and 4-cpm tachygastria waves and corresponding peaks in the RSA near 4 cpm (B1). Toward the end of the RSA, more peaks in the 1- to 2-cpm range are present. Thus, tachygastrias and bradygastrias developed after the water load in this patient. The percentage distribution of EGG power graphs show that power in the 3-cpm range is low during this EGG with water loading. On the other hand, bradygastria is at the upper limits of normal at baseline and 20 minutes after ingestion of water. There is a transient increase in tachygastria at the 10-minute period corresponding to B in the EGG rhythm strip and B1 in the RSA. By the 30-minute period, bradygastria percentages are increased. Thus, this is the pattern for a mixed gastric dysrhythmia after the water loading.

In some patients, tachygastria increases for longer periods of time, as shown in another example of a mixed dysrhythmia (Fig. 8.10). The EGG rhythm strip shows a 4- to 5-cpm tachygastria at 10 minutes (A) and a 2-cpm high-amplitude bradygastria at 30 minutes after the water load test. The RSA shows peaks at 4 and 5 cpm (A1) and 1- to 2-cpm peaks (B1). Few peaks at 3 cpm are seen. The mixed dysrhythmia pattern is also seen in the percentage distribution of power graphs. The distribution of EGG activity at baseline is within the normal ranges, but percentage of power in the tachygastria range is increased at 10 and 20 minutes after water loading and increased in the bradygastria range at 30 minutes.

The combinations of dysrhythmias are very erratic, and 3-cpm activity may be transiently normal in some patients with mixed dysrhythmias. Figure 8.11 shows the development of a mixed dysrhythmia after the water load test. The baseline EGG rhythm strip (A) shows several frequencies in the signal, including low-amplitude 2-cpm waves. The baseline RSA (A1) also shows a variety of frequency peaks. The patient ingested 530 ml of water. The EGG rhythm strip (B) from the 30-minute period after the water load shows an approximately 4-cpm

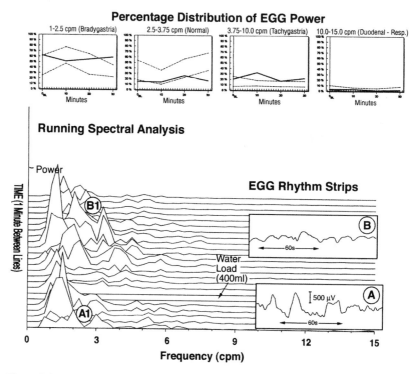

Figure 8.9. Mixed dysrhythmia with abnormal water load test. Electrogastrogram (EGG) rhythm strips, running spectral analysis (RSA), and percentage distribution of EGG power are shown from a patient with recurrent nausea and regurgitation. The baseline EGG shows 2-cpm activity (A). The RSA of baseline EGG activity shows large peaks at 1 to 2 cpm (A1). The EGG rhythm strip at (B) shows normal 3-cpm and 4-cpm tachygastria waves. Peaks in the RSA are seen near 3 cpm and 4 to 5 cpm (B1) corresponding to frequencies in the EGG waves. Toward the end of the RSA, more peaks in the 1- to 2-cpm range are present. The percentage distribution of EGG power shows very little 3-cpm activity during this EGG with water loading. Percentage of tachygastria increases at the 10 min. period corresponding to B in the EGG and B1 in the RSA. By the 30-minute time period, bradygastria percentages are increased.

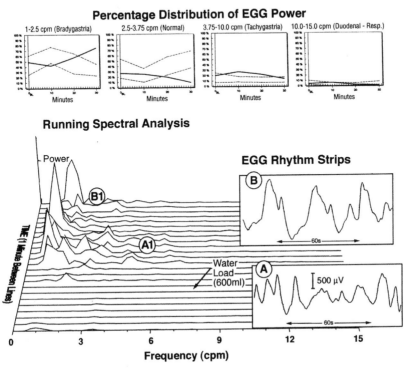

Percentage Distribution of EGG Power

1-2.5 cpm (Bradygastria)   2.5-3.75 cpm (Normal)   3.75-10.0 cpm (Tachygastria)   10.0-15.0 cpm (Duodenal - Resp.)

Minutes   Minutes   Minutes   Minutes

Running Spectral Analysis

Power

B1

A1

TIME (1 Minute Between Lines)

Water Load (600ml)

EGG Rhythm Strips

B

60s

A

500 µV

60s

0   3   6   9   12   15

Frequency (cpm)

Figure 8.10. Mixed dysrhythmia with normal water load test. Electrogastrogram (EGG) rhythm strips, running spectral analysis (RSA), and percentage distribution of EGG power are shown from a patient with dyspepsia. The baseline EGG rhythm strip is not shown. After 600 ml of water was ingested for the water load, the EGG rhythm strip shows a brief tachygastria at approximately 5 cpm (A). Small 5-cpm peaks are also seen in the RSA (A1). By the end of the recording, there are no 3-cpm peaks in the RSA, but peaks at 1 to 2 cpm are increased (B1). The EGG rhythm strip at (B) also shows the corresponding high-amplitude 2-cpm EGG waves. The percentage distribution of EGG power graphs show the EGG activity is within normal ranges ate baseline. After ingestion of the water load, the percentage of 3-cpm activity decreases while tachygastria increases transiently at 10 and 20 minutes, and bradygastria increases 30 minutes after the water load.

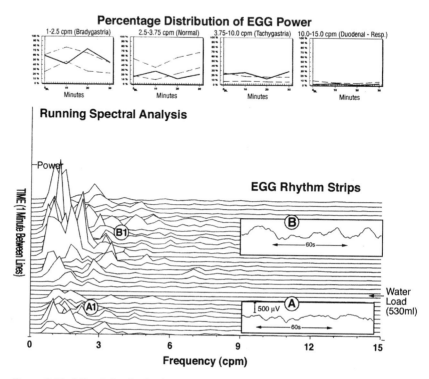

Figure 8.11. Mixed dysrhythmia with normal water load test. Electrogastrogram (EGG) rhythm strips, running spectral analysis (RSA), and percentage distribution of EGG power are shown from a patient with intermittent bloating and nausea. The baseline EGG rhythm strip (A) shows several frequencies, including 2-cpm low-amplitude waves (A). The baseline RSA (A1) also shows a variety of peaks. After the water load, a few peaks at 3 cpm developed in the RSA. The EGG rhythm strip shows approximately 4-cpm tachygastria (B) later in the recording and peaks are also seen at 4 cpm in the RSA (B1). By the end of the recording many peaks in the 1- to 2-cpm range are present. The percentage distribution of EGG power graphs show a brief increase in percentage 3-cpm activity after ingestion of water, increases in tachygastria at the 10- and the 30-minute periods and increased bradygastria activity 20 and 30 minutes after ingestion of the water.

tachygastria. Peaks in the RSA are also seen at 4 cpm (B1). By the end of the recording, there are many higher-power peaks in the 1- to 2-cpm range, as seen in previous RSAs of mixed dysrhythmias. The percentage distribution of EGG power graphs show the EGG activity is normal at baseline. The provocative water load test evoked a brief increase in 3-cpm activity at 10 minutes after the ingestion of water. There also is a slight increase in tachygastria at the 10- and 30-minute periods after the ingestion of water. Bradygastria activity is increased 20 and 30 minutes after ingestion of the water. Overall, this was a mixed gastric dysrhythmia.

Patients with GERD+ have a high incidence of mixed dysrhythmias. Figure 8.12 shows a mixed dysrhythmia in a patient with GERD and functional dyspepsia. Almost no increase in 3-cpm activity occurs at 10 minutes after the water load test, as shown in the EGG rhythm strip and the RSA. Tachygastria (4–5 cpm) developed at 20 minutes, as shown in the EGG rhythm strip (A) and the RSA (A1). Bradygastria activity increased at 30 minutes after ingestion of water as shown in the EGG rhythm strip (B) and the RSA (B1). The percentage distribution of EGG power graphs show the poor 3-cpm response to the normal water volume and the increased tachygastria activity at 20 minutes and increased bradygastria activity at 30 minutes after the water load test. This is a typical mixed dysrhythmia recorded from a patient with GERD and dyspepsia.

A subtle mixed dysrhythmia recorded from a patient with unexplained nausea is shown in Figure 8.13. Bradygastria is present in the EGG rhythm strip at baseline, and a transient increase in 3-cpm EGG activity is present after ingestion of water. However, tachygastria develops at 20 and 30 minutes after the water load, and then an increase in bradygastria occurs 30 minutes after the ingestion of water. The baseline EGG (A) shows some 3-cpm activity, but 2-cpm waves are also seen and the RSA at baseline shows corresponding frequency peaks at 2 and 3 cpm (A1). The patient ingested 500 ml of water as part of the water load test. The 5-cpm tachygastria is seen in the EGG signal (B). The dots identify the 5-cpm tachygastria waves. Peaks at 5 cpm are also seen in the RSA (B1). Toward the end of the recording, however, the tachygastria disappears and increased 1- to 2-cpm peaks develop in the EGG rhythm strip. (In C, the dotted lines outline the 1-cpm EGG waves.) Peaks at 1 cpm are seen in the RSA (C1). The percentage distribution of EGG power graphs show a brief increase in 3-cpm activity at 10 minutes after ingestion of the water but decreased 3-cpm activity

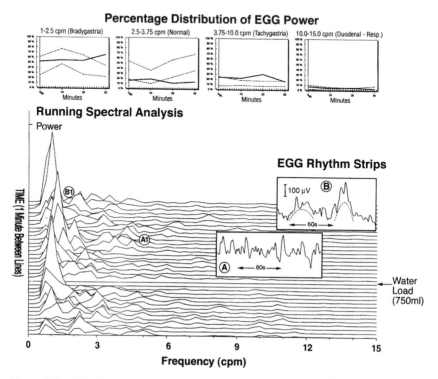

Figure 8.12. Mixed dysrhythmia with normal water load test. Electrogastrogram (EGG) rhythm strips, running spectral analysis (RSA), and percentage distribution of EGG power in a patient with esophageal reflux symptoms and dyspepsia. The EGG rhythm strip at (A) is recorded *after* ingestion of the water load and a 5- to 6-cpm tachygastria is seen; 4-, 5-, and 6-cpm peaks are also seen in the RSA at (A1). By the end of the recording, the EGG signal shows 1- to 2-cpm waves (B), and the RSA also shows peaks at 1 to 2 cpm (B1). The dotted line indicates the 1- to 2-cpm EGG waves on which higher-frequency waves are present. The percentage distribution of EGG power graphs show very poor 3-cpm response to the water load and increased percentage of tachygastria at 20 minutes after ingestion of water and increased bradygastria at 30 minutes after ingestion of water.

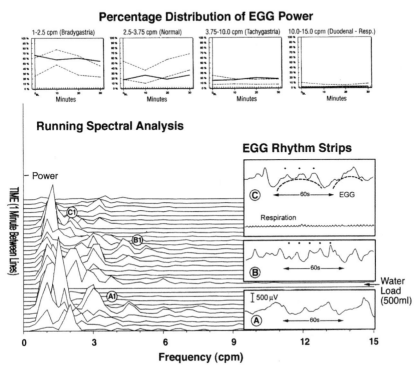

Figure 8.13. Mixed dysrhythmia with normal water load test. Electrogastrogram (EGG) rhythm strips, running spectral analysis (RSA), and percentage distribution of EGG power in a patient with recurrent nausea. The baseline EGG (A) shows some 3-cpm activity, but 2-cpm waves are also seen. The RSA at baseline shows corresponding frequency peaks at 2 and 3 cpm (A1). After the water load a transient 5-cpm tachygastria developed (B, note dots on 5-cpm waves) and 5 cpm peaks appear in the RSA (B1). Several 1- to 2-cpm waves are seen in the EGG rhythm strip (C) and in the RSA (C1) toward the end of the recording. The percentage distribution of EGG power graphs show a brief increase in 3-cpm activity at 10 minutes after ingestion of the water, but below-normal activity thereafter. Slight increase in tachygastria percentage was seen at 20 minutes and an increase in the bradygastria is seen at 30 min. after ingestion of water.

207

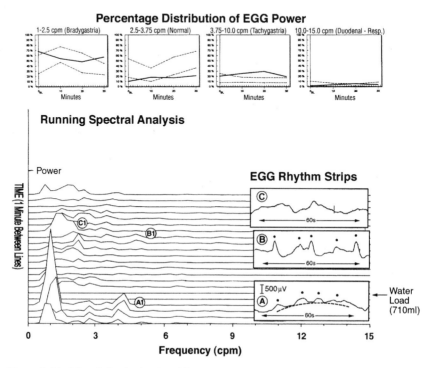

Figure 8.14. Mixed dysrhythmia with normal water load test. Electrogastrogram (EGG) rhythm strips, running spectral analysis (RSA), and percentage distribution of EGG power in a patient with reflux and nausea. The baseline EGG shows a long duration bradygastria wave at 1 cpm (see dotted lines) with 4 smaller waves (black dots) "riding" the larger wave (A). The baseline RSA shows peaks at 4 cpm (A1) as well as 1- to 2-cpm peaks, reflecting the frequencies in the EGG signal. The patient ingested 710 ml of water. A 5- to 6-cpm tachygastria (see black dots) developed as shown in the EGG rhythm strip (B); corresponding small peaks in the RSA are seen at 5 cpm (B1). There are 1- to 2-cpm waves in the EGG signal (C) and 1- to 2-cpm peaks in the RSA (C1) and reflect the minutes of EGG signal towards the end of the recording.

208

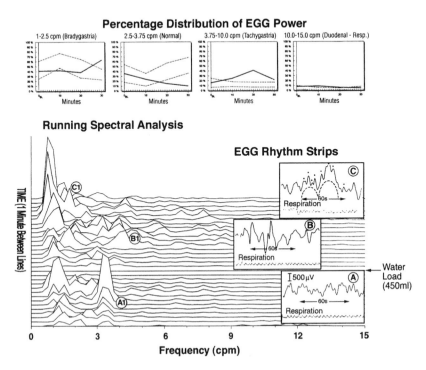

Figure 8.15. Mixed dysrhythmia with normal water load test. Electrogastrogram (EGG) rhythm strips, running spectral analysis (RSA), and percentage distribution of EGG power in a patient with nausea. The baseline EGG this shows 3-cpm activity (A). Respiration (RESP) is also shown. Peaks at 3.5 cpm are seen in the RSA at baseline (A1). Very little 3-cpm activity is present after ingestion of water, but 4-cpm and 6-cpm activity develop in the EGG signal at (B) and are shown as 4 and 6 cpm peaks in the RSA at (B1). By the end of the recording, there are 1–2 cpm EGG waves (C) (outlined by dotted lines) and corresponding high power peaks at 1–2 in the RSA (C1). Faster waves at about 8 cpm are carried on the bradygastria waves (C). The percentage distribution of EGG power shows progressive loss of percentage 3-cpm activity after ingestion of water, increased tachygastria at 20 and 30 minutes and increased bradygastria at 30 minutes after water ingestion.

209

thereafter. A slight increase in tachygastria percentage was present at 20 minutes, and an increase in the bradygastria activity was present at 30 minutes after ingestion of water.

An EGG with a 1-cpm gently curving wave in the baseline rhythm strip is shown in Figure 8.14. Four smaller waves (indicated by the four dots) are superimposed on this 1-cpm wave, which is outlined by the dotted line. The RSA also shows peaks at baseline at 1 and 4 cpm (A1). This patient ingested 710 ml of water, but no 3-cpm peaks are seen in the RSA after the water load. Several peaks in the RSA are seen in the tachygastria (B1) and bradygastria (C1) range after ingestion of water. The EGG rhythm strip at (B) shows a 5-cpm tachygastria that corresponds to the peaks at 5 cpm in the RSA (B1). The bradygastria that developed later as shown in (C) corresponds to the 1- to 2-cpm peaks in the RSA (C1). Thus, this is a mixed dysrhythmia response to ingestion of water.

Figure 8.15 shows a mixed dysrhythmia pattern with normal 3-cpm peaks at baseline but poor 3-cpm response to the water load. The baseline EGG shows 3-cpm activity (A). Peaks at 3.5 cpm are seen in the RSA at baseline (A1). The patient ingested 450 ml of water during the water load test. Very little 3-cpm activity was seen after the ingestion of water. Both 4- and 5-cpm tachygastrias (B) occur initially after the water load, and prominent 1- to 2-cpm EGG waves occur later. By the end of the recording, there were increased waves in the EGG from 1 to 2 cpm (C) and high-power peaks at 1 to 2 cpm in the RSA (C1). These bradygastria waves also carry other waves at faster frequencies of approximately 8 cpm. Small peaks in the RSA are present at 8 to 9 cpm after the water load. The respiration rate is 16 breaths per minute. The percentage distribution of EGG power was normal at baseline, but progressive loss of 3-cpm activity occurred after the ingestion of water and tachygastria increased at 20 and 30 minutes and bradygastria increased at 30 minutes after water ingestion.

References

1. Koch KL: Electrogastrography. In: Schuster M, Crowell M, and Koch KL, eds. *Atlas of Gastrointestinal Motility.* Hamilton, Ontario, Canada: BC Decker;2002.
2. Hinder RA, Kelley KA: Human gastric pacesetter potential: site of origin, spread, and response to gastric transection and proximal vagotomy. *Am J Surg* 1997;133:29–33.

3. Smout AJPM, van der Schee EJ, Grashuis JL: What is measured in electrogastrography? *Dig Dis Sci* 1980;25:179–187.

4. You CH, Chey WY, Lee KY, et al: Gastric and small intestinal myoelectric dysrhythmia associated with chronic intractable nausea and vomiting. *Ann Intern Med* 1981;95:449–451.

5. Familoni BO, Bowes KL, Kingma WJ, et al: Can transcutaneous recordings detect gastric electrical abnormalities? *Gut* 1991;32:141–146.

6. Koch KL, Stern RM, Vasey M, et al: Gastric dysrhythmias and nausea of pregnancy. *Dig Dis Sci* 1990;35:961–968.

7. Amaris MA, Sanmiguel CP, Sadowski DC, et al: Electrical activity from colon overlaps with normal gastric electrical activity in cutaneous recordings. *Dig Dis Sci* 2002;47:2480–2485.

8. Verhagan MAMT, van Schelven AJ, Samsom M, et al: Pitfalls of the analysis of electrogastrographic recordings. *Gastroenterology* 1999;117:453–460.

9. Koch KL, Hong S-P, Xu L: Reproducibility of gastric myoelectrical activity and the water load test in patients with dysmotility-like dyspepsia symptoms and in control subjects. *J Clin Gastroenterol* 2000;31:125–129.

10. Parkman HP, Miller MA, Trate D, et al: Electrogastrography in gastric emptying scintigraphy are complimentary for assessment of dyspepsia. *J Clin Gastroenterol* 1997;24:214–219.

11. Koch KL, Stern RM, Stewart WR, et al: Gastric emptying and gastric myoelectrical activity in patients with symptomatic diabetic gastroparesis: Effects of long-term domperidone treatment. *Am J Gastroenterol* 1989;84:1069–1075.

12. Brzana RJ, Bingaman S, Koch KL: Gastric myoelectrical activity in patients with gastric outlet obstruction and idiopathic gastroparesis. *Am J Gastroenterol* 1998;93:1083–1089.

13. Koch KL, Stern RM, Vasey M, et al: Gastric dysrhythmias and nausea of pregnancy. *Dig Dis Sci* 1987;32:919.

14. Sun WM, Smout AJPM, Malbert C, et al: Relationship between surface electrogastrography and antropyloric pressures. *Am J Physiol* 1995;268:G424–G430.

15. Lind JF, Duthie HL, Schlegel JF, et al: Motility of the gastric fundus. *Am J Physiol* 1961;201:197–202.

16. Verhagon MAMT, Luijk HD, Samson M, et al: Effect of meal temperature on the frequency of gastric electrical activity. *Neurogastroenterology* 1998;10:175–181.

17. Lin HC, Zho X-T, Chung B, et al: Frequency of gastric pacesetter potential depends on volume and site of distention. *Am J Physiol* 1996;270:G470–G475.

18. Ladabaum U, Brown MB, Pan W, et al: Effects of nutrients and serotonin 5-HT_3 antagonism on symptoms evoked by distal gastric distention in humans. *Am J Physiol* 2001;280:G201–G208.

19. San Miguel CP, Mintchev MP, Bowes KL: Dynamics of level of randomness of electrogastrograms can be indicative of gastric electrical uncoupling in dogs. *Dig Dis Sci* 1999;44:523–528.
20. Ordog T, Baldo M, Danko R, et al: Plasticity of electrical pacemaking by interstitial cells of Cajal and gastric dysrhythmias in W/W^v mutant mice. *Gastroenterology* 2002;123:2028–2040.
21. Pezzolla F, Riezzo G, Maselli MA, et al: Electrical activity recorded from abdominal surface after gastrectomy or colectomy in humans. *Gastroenterology* 1989;97:313–320.
22. Amaris MA, Sanmiguel CP, Sadowski DC, et al: Electrical activity from colon overlaps with normal gastric electrical activity in cutaneous recordings. *Dig Dis Sci* 2002;47:2480–2485.
23. Koch KL, Xu L, Noar M: Gastric myoelectrical and emptying activity in patients with gastroesophageal reflux disease (GERD) and dysmotility-like functional dyspepsia (GERD+): effect of water load test. *Am J Gastroenterol* 2001;96:526.

9

The Future and Electrogastrography

The 3–cycles per minute (cpm) gastric pacesetter potential is a fundamental electrical phenomenon of the stomach. This low-frequency biorhythm is the basis for normal neuromuscular function of the stomach. In regard to the origins and the various neural and hormonal influences that affect the 3-cpm rhythm, many mysteries remain. Ongoing and future inquiries into the very nature of rhythmicity will provide deeper understanding of gastric myoelectrical activity and the electrical activity detected in the electrogastrogram (EGG). The role of knockout mice that lack interstitial cells of Cajal will be increasingly important in understanding the crucial role of rhythmic electrical events in normal and abnormal neuromuscular function of the stomach. These and other animal studies will also continue to help clinicians understand the deficits in gastric neuromuscular function caused by electrical dysrhythmias.

A delicate balance maintains normal 3-cpm activity. Stomach electrical rhythmicity is rather unstable during fasting, for example, compared with the rhythmic 3-cpm electrical events and contractile events that occur in the postprandial period. What mechanisms produce these fasting and postprandial electrical changes? Are neural or hormonal circuits most critical? Are extrinsic or intrinsic nerves the most important? Studies of fasting and postprandial EGG activity may offer insights into sensations of hunger and satiety.

The EGG signal is responsive to brain–gut interactions such as the cephalic-vagal reflex. Sham feeding studies with healthy subjects indicated that the sight, smell, and taste of food significantly increased 3-cpm activity. However, in subjects who indicated that the sham feeding experience was disgusting, no increase in 3-cpm activity occurred in this situation. Future studies of patients with eating disorders such as bulimia or anorexia nervosa using EGG recording methods may reveal new insights into the pathophysiology of eating disorders and be of value in monitoring the progress of treatment.

Different EGG patterns induced by different meals reflect the different gastric neuromuscular work required to receive, mix, and empty the specific meal. Characteristics of the EGG signal from frequency to amplitude may also correlate with perceptions of stomach fullness, hunger, or satiety. Future studies of the EGG may define these relationships and provide important clues regarding the contribution of the stomach to perceptions of hunger and satiety, perceptions that are important in regard to the development of obesity.

Gastroenterologists use EGG recordings to diagnose gastric dysrhythmias in different and complex cases where unexplained upper gastrointestinal symptoms persist. The future will bring EGG technology into the offices of the internist and family physician. EGG recordings will assist these physicians in the diagnosis of unexplained dyspepsia symptoms, much like electrocardiographic (ECG) technology is used in the office to diagnose cardiovascular abnormalities in patients with palpitations or chest symptoms. The process of diagnosing cardiovascular symptoms frequently begins with an ECG recording to determine if a cardiac dysrhythmia or other electrical abnormality is present. Similarly, a noninvasive high-quality EGG recording with standard provocative test will provide a diagnosis of gastric dysrhythmia (or normal 3-cpm myoelectrical activity) and aid the physician in the diagnosis and management of patients with unexplained nausea and dyspepsia symptoms.

Future studies will help us to determine whether gastric dysrhythmias reflect primarily interstitial cells of Cajal disorders versus neurogenic disorders versus disorders that affect primarily smooth muscle. Many patients will have combinations of injury and dysfunction of these elements. EGG frequencies in patients with myogenic disorders are more irregular and chaotic compared with patients with neurogenic disorders. Such differences will be clarified and provide additional help with selecting drug or device therapies for these patients.

Future studies will continue to indicate that gastric dysrhythmias are the disorder and that restoration of normal 3-cpm EGG activity is associated with resolution of symptoms such as nausea, upper abdominal discomfort, bloating, and uncomfortable fullness and early satiety. These symptoms are now simply categorized as *functional dyspepsia.* In the future, the gastric dysrhythmias such as tachygastria and bradygastria will be treated with a variety of specific antiarrhythmic therapies. The treatment of such symptoms will then be placed on an objective and rational basis, preventing unnecessary testing, unnecessary use of ineffective drugs, and more efficacious and predictable treatment of symptoms. Thus, new drug development based on the correction of an objective gastric abnormality—gastric dysrhythmias—is an exciting use of EGG recordings.

The EGG will also be useful in quantifying the efficacy of pharmaceutical or device treatments for nausea, bloating, and other dyspepsia symptoms that are due to gastric neuromuscular dysfunction. Treatments in the future may also involve alternative medications in the form of herbs and acustimulation, or acupuncture therapies. Treatment with antiarrhythmic or prokinetic drugs, or alternative therapies may take an unknown amount of time to restore normal gastric myoelectrical function. Improvement in myoelectrical activity may precede full resolution of symptoms. Improvement in the EGG pattern may indicate that the clinician should continue current therapy. On the other hand, no improvement in the EGG after a specific therapy may be grounds to try a different therapeutic approach.

Biofeedback is another form of therapy that may be used in the future to help restore normal 3-cpm activity. Biofeedback has been used successfully in the treatment of fecal incontinence, but it has not been used systematically to reduce upper gastrointestinal symptoms. The 3-cpm EGG rhythm may be strengthened if used in conjunction with standard biofeedback techniques. In preliminary studies with healthy subjects, we were able to show that biofeedback methods could be used to increase 3-cpm activity in healthy subjects. Thus, biofeedback techniques may be helpful in patients who have gastric dysrhythmias by improving 3-cpm activity, decreasing the gastric dysrhythmias, and decreasing upper gastrointestinal symptoms.

Gastric electrical stimulation and gastric pacemakers are technologies that will be used more frequently in the future for the treatment of severe gastroparesis. As a neuromuscular organ, the stomach has many electrical and contractile attributes that are similar to those of the heart. Thus, it is reasonable to anticipate that some form of electrical pacing or stimulation will benefit many patients with gastric dysrhythmias and gastroparesis. To date, the present pacemaking and electrical stimulating parameters have not consistently produced improvement in gastric electrical activity or emptying. Pulse width, duration, and frequency of electrical stimulation are still in the early phases of study, and optimal stimulation parameters have yet to be defined. The number and location of stimulating electrodes are other important variables that will be refined in the future. In the realm of cardiac diseases, the pathophysiology of a patient's symptoms are understood because tests of cardiac electrical function, contractile function, and the studies of valves and coronary arteries are performed and interpreted. In an analogous fashion, the patient's upper gastrointestinal symptoms are better understood and therapies are placed on a more rational basis when electrogastrogram patterns and gastric emptying rates are determined. These tests will also define baseline neuromuscular characteristics that can be compared with studies performed weeks and months after gastric pacemaking therapy commences.

In addition to hospital-, office-, and laboratory-based EGG recordings, the future will provide further improvements in technology that will allow the recording of ambulatory EGG signals. We have been involved in studies of EGG recordings from astronauts in space in an attempt to learn more about gastric myoelectrical events during space motion sickness. Ambulatory EGG recording would provide continuous 24-hour information about gastric myoelectrical activity and upper gastrointestinal symptoms, which may aid in the diagnosis of patients with episodic symptoms.

A substantial body of scientific knowledge exists that supports the use of EGG recording techniques in a wide variety of interesting medical and nonmedical diagnosis of gastric dysrhythmias and to record changes in gastric myoelectrical activity in diverse situations. With attention to technique and methods, high-quality EGG signals can be recorded. When high-quality EGG signals are analyzed by computer, new insights are revealed and quantitative data can be derived for clinical and experimental purposes. It is hoped that the *Handbook of Electrogastrography* provides a foundation for those clinicians and researchers interested in the physiology of gastric myoelectrical activity and the applications of electrogastrography.

Index

....